MOLECULAR BIOLOGY FOR ADVANCED LEARNERS

1st Edition

- Mr. M. Pradsad Naidu
PhD Scholar
Dr NTR University of Health Sciences
Vijayawada
Andhra Pradesh, India.

- Mr. G. Amar Nagesh Kumar
PhD Scholar
Dr NTR University of Health Sciences
Vijayawada
Andhra Pradesh, India.

- Dr S. V, Prasad, Ph.D.,
Department of Biology,
STPM Govt. Institute Advanced Studies in Education,
Nellore, Andhra Pradesh, India.

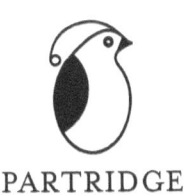

PARTRIDGE

To order additional copies of this book, contact
Partridge India
000 800 10062 62
orders.india@partridgepublishing.com

www.partridgepublishing.com/india

Contents

Preface

"Molecular Biology for Advanced Learners" textbook was planned by me and executed by other two authors as well, essentially for the students of medical, dental, pharmacy, paramedical, and allied biological sciences. This book gives core information and offers a quick and easy exposition of concepts when time is at a premium, especially before the examination.

This book is different from the books already available in the market by different ways. For example this book is having new figures, new information regarding molecular biology, which is very easy to remember and figures are self explanatory.

Molecular biology techniques have been made more illustrative and simple which is not present in undergraduate molecular biology books. This book can also be used profitably for entrance examination of MSc, M.Phil., B.Sc, MLT, Nursing, BPT, B.Pharmacy., in disciplines such as biochemistry, molecular biology, biotechnology, genetics and also for other life sciences competitive examinations.

We are extra-cautious in presenting the matter in easy and lucid language. A glossary has been made in the end of the book so as to enable the students to learn the meaning and origin of the words used in the text. The diagrams are specially designed for clearly and simplicity.

I conclude this preface with the words of **Sri. K.Sreenivasa Rao** "The fortunate ones are thrice blessed: the first blessing is to have a preffession that can lead to organized discoveries. The second blessing is to share these discoveries with many colleagues. The third blessing is to make discoveries that improve the quality of life" I would like to thank **the Dr. K. Chandra Mouli** Krishna, Assistant Professor Department of Pharmacology for their help & cooperation extended during the study.

I express my deepest gratitude to my research guide, **Dr. Duggirala Rajarajeswari** M.D, Associate professor, Department of Biochemistry, for her support to my PhD research work. Last but not the least I sincerely thank my parents Mr. M. Krishnaiah and Mrs. M. Bala for their unconditional love and support without which I could not have accomplished this book.

M Prasad Naidu

Scientists

1869 Isolation of DNA for the first time by Friedrich Miescher

1881 Edward Zacharias showed chromosomes are composed of nuclein.

1899 Nuclein renamed as Nucleic acid by Richard Altmann.

1900 Elucidation of chemical structures of all 20 amino acids

1902 - Emil Hermann Fischer showed amino acids are building blocks of proteins. Postulated: Properties of proteins are defined by amino acid composition and sequence and wins Nobel Prize.

1911 Thomas Hunt Morgan discovers genes on chromosomes are the discrete units of heredity.

1911 Discovery of RNA by Pheobus Aaron Theodore Lerene.

1928 F. Grifth – found the phenomenon of transformation in bacteria.

1934 M. Schlesinger – demonstrated that the bacteriophages are made of protein and DNA.

1941 G.W. Beadle and E.L. Tatum – Published their classical study on the biochemical genetics of Neurospora.

1943 – 1947 Leloir and Munoz – demonstrated oxidation of fatty acids in cell-free systems.

1944 Ostwald T. Avery, Colin m. Macleod and Maclyn McCarty- demonstrated that DNA is genetic material also bacterial transformation is caused by DNA.

1947 *By a*pplying Chagraff's rules and the X-ray image from Rosalind Franklin, Crick constructed (a "tinkertoy" model showing) the double helix. (*"In 1947 Crick knew no organic chemistry and practically no biology or crystallography"*) Their

1953 *Nature* paper: *"It has not escaped our notice that the specific pairing we have postulated immediately suggests a possible copying mechanism for the genetic material."*

1948 A. Boivin, R. Vendrely and C. Vendrely: Showed that in different cells of an organism the quantity of DNA for each haploid set of chromosome is constant.

1950 Isolation t-RNA by Mahlon Bush Hoagland.

1952 Genes made from DNA by Alfred Hershey and Martha Chase.

1950 – 1953 Erwin Chargaff – discovered the base equivalences in Deoxyribonucleic acid.

1953 James D. Watson and Francis Harry Comptom Crick – proposed the double -helix structure of DNA, based on x-ray diffraction patterns. (Waton, Crick and Wilkins, Nobel Laureates, 1962).

1955 – 1957 Arthur Kornberg and Severo Ochoa – synthesis of DNA by Kornberg and RNA by Ochoa artificially outside of cells, i.e., in vitro (Nobel Laureates, 1959).

1956 George Emil Palade demonstrated the site of enzymes synthesis in the cytoplasm is made on RNA organelles known as Ribosomes.

1956 A. Gierer and G. Schramm – found that RNA is the genetic material of TMV.

1957 H. Fraenkel – Contrat and B. Singer – resolved RNA from the protein of TMV viruses, produced hybrid RNA viruses and confirmed the view that RNA is the genetic material of certain viruses.

1957 Arthur Kornberg – discovered DNA polymerase, which is used to produce labelled DNA probes.

1958 Demonstration of DNA replication by a semi conservative mechanism by Meselson and Stahl.

1958 G. Beadle and E. Tatum – Nobel Laureates, 1959 for their contribution in biochemical genetics of fungus.

1959 Isolation of single-stranded DNA from a small virus φ-X-174 by R.L. Sinsheimer which attacks E. coli. S. Ochoa; A. Kornberg – won the Nobel Prize for artificial synthesis of nucleic acids.

1961 Marshall W. Neirenberg and J.H. Matthaei – deciphered the Genetic Code (Nirenberg, Nobel Laureate, 1968).

1961 Francois Jacob and Jacques Monod – presented operon model for the regulation of gene activity (Nobel Laureates, 1965).

1962 J. Watson and F. Crick; M. Wilkens – received Novel Prize for the discovery of molecular nature of DNA.

1963 J.P. Waller – reported that about one-half of all proteins in E. coli cells have the amino acid Methionine in the N-terminal position.

1963 John Cairns – discovered the existence of circular DNA in a bacterium.

1964 K.A. Marcker and F. Sanger – deciphered a peculiar aminoacyl-t-RNA in E.coli called N-formyl-methionyl – tRNA and reported that this molecule may play a vital role in chain elongation mechanisms. R.W. Holley and his colleagues gave a detailed structure of alanyl tRNA (tRNA ^{ala}) from yeast. Doty – discovered renaturation of DNA.

1965 Robert W. Holley et al – deciphered the base sequence of a nucleic acid (Nobel Laureate, 1968). H. Wallace and M.L. Birnstiel – isolated r- RNA genes in Xenopus.

1965 F. Jacob., A. Lwoff, and J. Monod – awarded Nobel Prize for the discovery of mechanism of protein synthesis in viruses.

1966 Marshall H. Nirenbnerg, Severo Ochoa and Arthur Kornberg – elucidated the Genetic Code.

1966 Gilbert and Muller. Hill – isolation of the lac repressor.

1967 Waclow Szybalski – demonstrated that only one strand of DNA is transcribed.

1968 Glomset – postulated the theory of reverse cholesterol transport where HDL is involved in the return of cholesterol to the liver.

1968 R.W. Holley; H.G. Khorana and M.W. Nirenberg – awarded Nobel Prize for deciphering the genetic code.

1969 A.D. Hershey, M. Delbruck and S.E. Luria – shared Nobel Prize for their contributions to replication and recombination in bacteriophages (viruses). Britten and Davidson postulated the gene-battery model for regulation of protein synthesis in eukaryotes.

1970 Howard Temin and David Baltimore – (Nobel Laureates, 1957 for the discovery of RNA directed DNA polymerase (or) reverse transcriptase which is present in the core of virus particle called rous sarcoma virus. Demonstrated the synthesis of DNA on RNA template tumor viruses.

1970 Knippers: Kornberg and Gefter; Moses and Richardson isolated DNA-polymerase-II enzyme.

1972 Mertz and Davis demonstrated that cohesive termini of cleaved DNA could be covalently sealed with E.coli DNA ligase and were able to produce r-DNA molecules.

1972 Cohen et al., reported for the first time about the cloning of DNA by using plasmid as vector.

1972 R. Porter; G.M. Edelman awarded Nobel Prize for the discovery of chemical structure of antibodies. C.B. Anfinsen; S. Moore and W.H. Stein received Nobel Prize for the discovery of chemical structure and activity of ribonuclease.

1973 Cohen, Chang, Boyer and Helling – demonstrated the first DNA cloning experiments.

1973 S.H. Kim deciphered 3D-structure of t-RNA.

1975 E.M. Southern developed Southern blotting technique for analyzing the related genes in a DNA restriction fragment. D. Pribnow deciphered Pribnow box or minus ten sequence in E. coli genome.

1976 W. Gilbert, A. Maxam, and Frederick Sanger – developed methods for determination of base sequence in DNA (Gilbert and Sanger, Nobel Laureates, 1980).

1976 Kim, Rich and Klug – described the detailed 3D – structure of t-RNA determined by x-ray diffraction methods.

1977 P.A. Sharp and R.J. Roberts found split genes of adenovirus. D.S. Hogness, I.B. David and N. Davidson reported split genes for 28 S r-RNA in Drosophila. P. Chambon, P. Leder and R.A. Flavell studied split genes of B'globin, ovalbumin and t-RNA. Itakura et al., produced human insulin (humalin) by recombinant technology.

1977 Phillip Sharp and Richard Roberts reported that pre-mRNA is processed by the excision of introns and exons are spliced together.

1978 – 79 W. Gilbert for the first time used the terms exons and introns (for split genes).

1978 Hinnen et al., for the first time explained the transformation of yeast (Saccharomyces cervisae) with the help of plasmid of E.coli.

1979 Khorana synthesized a biologically functional gene. Alwine et al., developed northern blotting technique. (mRNA bands transferred from the gel onto chemically reactive paper). Towbin et al., introduced the western blotting technique to find out the newly encoded protein by a transformed cell.

1980 Fredrick Sanger got Nobel Prize (2nd time) for deciphering complete sequence of 5400 nucleotides of single stranded DNA of ϕ x 174 bacteriophage.

1982 A. Klug was awarded Nobel Prize for providing 3D- structure of t-RNA.

1982 R.D. Palmiter and R.L. Brinter produced transgenic mice by genetic engineering method.

1983 Marilyn Kozak proposed the scanning hypothesis for initiation of translation by eukaryotic ribosomes.

1982 – 1984 Sidney Altman and Thomas R. Cech – found RNA catalysis (Nobel Laureates 1989).

1984 Schwartz and Cantor – invented pulsed field gel electrophoresis (separation of very large DNA molecules).

1985 Kary B Mullis – invented the polymerase chain reaction (PCR), (amplification of tiny amounts of DNA).

1984-86 Alec Jeffreys discovered DNA finger printing.

1986 Leroy Hood: Developed automated sequencing mechanism.

1986 Human Genome Initiative announced

1987 S. Tonegawa (Nobel Laureate) produced a large variety of antibodies by a mode of rearrangement of DNA sequences of mammalian immunoglobulin genes.

1988 J.W. Black, G.B. Elion and G.H. Hitchings(Nobel Laureates1988) for formulating drugs such as 6- mercaptopurine and thioguanine (which inhibits DNA synthesis and cell division). This proved effective in cancer chemotherapy.

1989 T. Cech and S. Altman won the Nobel Prize for showing enzymatic role of ribozymes.

1990 The 15 year Human Genome project is launched by congress.

1991 Dr. Lalji Singh at CCMB, Hyderabad has introduced a new technique of DNA fingerprinting by using BKM-DNA probe (BKM = banded krait minor satellite).

1992 Edwin G. Krebs and Edmond H. Fisher received Nobel Prize for the pioneering work on "reversible protein phosphorylation as a biological regulator mechanism." Phosphorylation of proteins is shown to affect transcription, translation, cell division and many other cellular processes.

1993 M.J. Chamberlain postulated the inchworm model for elongation of transcript of DNA template.

1995 Moderate-resolution maps of chromosomes 3, 11, 12, and 22 maps published (These maps provide the locations of "markers" on each chromosome useful in locating genes easier).

1995 John Craig Venter: Bacterial genomes sequenced for the first time.

1996 First eukaryotic genome-yeast-sequenced.

1997 E. Coli sequenced.

1998 The genome of Caenorhabditis elegans completely sequenced.

1999 For the first time human chromosome (number 22) sequenced.

2000 The euchromatic portion of the Drosophila melanogaster genome completely sequenced.

2001 International Human Genome Sequencing first draft of the sequence of the human genome published.

April 2003 Genome of Human Project Completed. Genome of mouse is sequenced.

April 2004 Genome of Rat sequenced.

Chapter 1
NUCLEIC ACIDS

Nucleic acids are the important molecules as, their primary structure includes a code or set of directions by which they can duplicate themselves leading to synthesis of proteins. The proteins synthesized - most of which are enzymes - ultimately governs the metabolic activities of the cell. In 1953, Watson, an American biologist, and Crick, an English biologist, proposed the double helical model for DNA. This development set the stage for a new technology for chemical and biological investigation. The two main events in the life of a cell - dividing to make exact copies of themselves, and manufacturing proteins - both rely on blueprints coded in our genes. Nucleic acids are polymers of nucleotide mono phosphate residues. Nucleotides are joined by phosphodiester bonds between the OH on position three of the ribose sugar of specific nucleotide and the phosphate group on position 5 of another nucleotide. Each poly nucleotide has two ends (primes); 3` prime which contains the OH group and the 5` prime which possesses the PO_4 group.

The Nucleic Acids are divided into two categories namely RNA & DNA. In different organisms the genetic information is stored either within the DNA or the RNA.
Examples: Bacterial Viruses (Bacteriophages) ϕ x 174, λ, T_2, T_4, have DNA. F_2, Ms_2, R_{17}, & Q_β have RNA as genetic Material.

Animal Viruses
Simian Virus 40, Mouse polyoma & Rabbit papilloma, Herpes simplex, adenovirus have DNA. Rous sarcoma in fowl, poliomyelitis, influenza, Reo virus have RNA, as genetic material.

Plant Viruses
T.M.V. & Tomatobushy stunt have RNA
The nucleic acids are polynucleotide esters made up of Nucleoside & the phosphate group, the nucleosides are further made up of pentose sugar and Nitrogenous base.

Nucleic acid is a polymer of nucleotide and Nitrogenous base. Nucleic acid Pentose in RNA is ribose while in DNA, it is 2' Deoxy ribose. But the pentose occur in the nucleotide in their β – furanase form. The PO_4 group is esterified usually at 5' position & in the cell pH has a –ve charge. The Nitrogenous bases are linked to the 1' carbon by N-glycosyl linkage.

Nucleotide is composed of Nucleoside + phosphate group. The nucleotides are formed by the esterification of phosphoric acid on the nucleoside. Since the ribonucleosides have 3 free 'OH' groups 3 possible ribonucleoside mono phosphates can be formed.

Nucleoside is made up of pentose sugar +Nitrogenous base. A nucleoside is formed by the combination of pentose sugar and purine & pyrimidine base, where the bases are linked by N-glycosidic linkage to the 1' carbon. The linkage occurs at 9th position in purine, where as it occurs at 1st position of base in pyrimidine

Nucleoside and nucleotide

Nucleic acids are polymers of mononucleotides they are by 3' and 5'phosphor diester bonds

Nucleoside --- Base + Sugar

Nucleotide --- Base + sugar + phosphate
          (Phosphorylatednucleoside).

Nitrogenous bases are the derivatives of 2-parent heterocyclic compounds namely pyrimidine & purine.

BASES Nitrogenous bases are heterocyclic compounds. They are mainly of two types:

Purines	Pyrimidines
Adenine	Cytosine
Guanine	Thymine
	Uracil

Figure 1.1 Purines and Pyrimidines structures

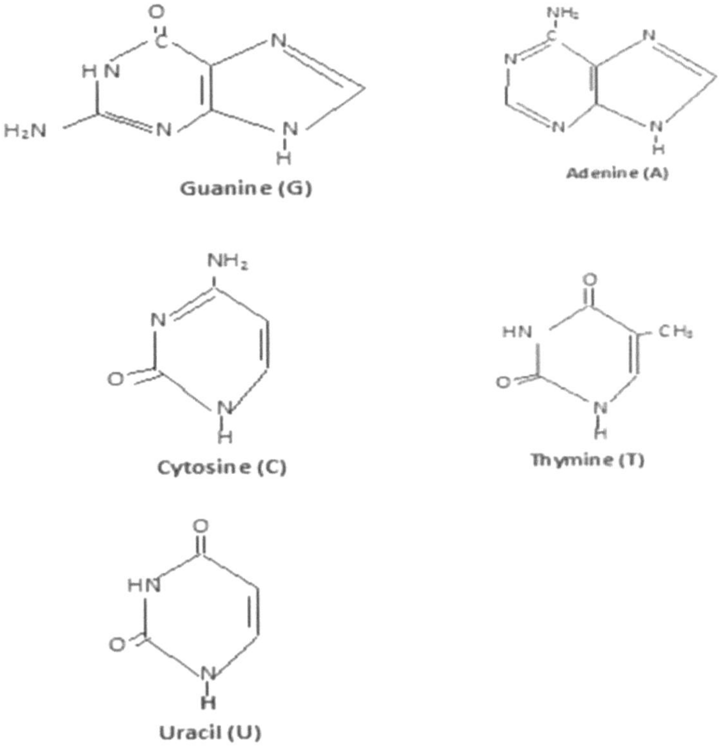

Guanine (G)

Adenine (A)

Cytosine (C)

Thymine (T)

Uracil (U)

Purines are numbered in ***anticlockwise*** direction in pyrimidine ring and clockwise direction in imidazole ring. Purines are two-ringed nitrogen compounds. These are numbered in anticlock direction.

ADENINE - 6 – amino purine
GUANINE – 2-amino 6 oxy purine
Pyrimidine: These are single ringed nitrogen compounds. Pyrimidines are numbered in clock wise direction. Apart from these some methylated minor bases occur. In some viral DNAs methylated or glycosylated minor bases occur. Such bases have specific roles as signals.

Figure 1.2 Purine structure

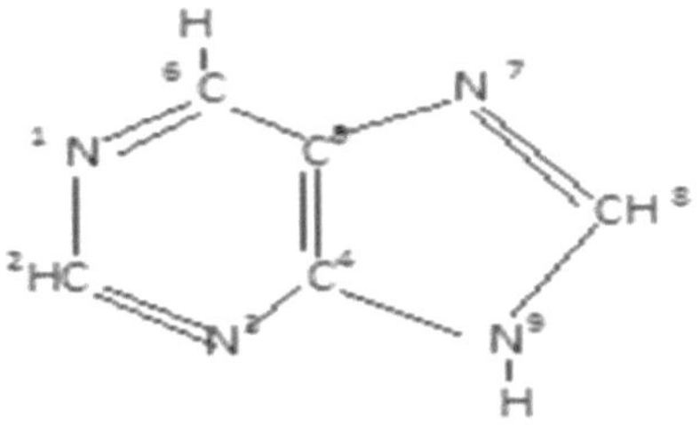

The pyrimidine bases usually undergo ketoenoltautemerium. Pyrimidines are numbered in ***clockwise*** direction Cytosine and thiamine are commonly found in DNA Cytosine and Uracil are found in RNA.

Tautomerism: **Figure 1.3 Pyrimidine structure**

Tautomerism forms of purines and pyrimidines.

The existence of a molecule in α keto(Lactam) and enol (lactim) form is known as tautomerism. Tautomerism is exhibited by the heterocyclic rings of purines and pyrimidines with oxo (-C-) functional groups.

The purine – guanine and pyrimidines – cytosine thymine and Uracil exhibit tautomerism.

Pentoses of Nucleic Acids

- The five carbon monosaccharide's (pentoses) are found in the nucleic acid structure.
- Pentose in RNA is D-ribose and DNA is D- deoxyribose.
- Deoxyribose and ribose differ in C_2.
- D-deoxyribose has an oxygen less than Ribose.

The carbons of sugars are represented with an associated prime (') for differentiation. Thus the pentose carbons are 1' to 5'. The pentoses are bound to nitrogenous bases by β – N- glycosidic bonds. The purine ring (N^9) is bound to pentose sugar (C_1) through an a covalent bond.

In pyrimidine nucleosides, the glycosidic linkage is between N^1 of a pyrimidine and C_2 of pentose. The hydroxyl groups of adenosine are esterified with phosphates to produce at 5' and 3' monophosphate.5' – Hydroxyl is the most common estimation hence 5' is usually omitted while writing nucleotide names. Thus AMP represents adenosine 5' monophosphate however for adenosine 3'-monophosphate the abbreviation 3'- AMP is used.

Phosphodiester bond: It involves two ester – O - bonds.
Many nucleotides are linked together to form a polynucl2leotide chain.

Two nucleotides are joined by d-phosphodiester bond. Phosphodiester Bond is formed between the C_3 of sugar of one nucleotide and the phosphate component at the 5' position of another nucleotide.

Major bases in nucleic acids:

- Both DNA and RNA contain purines like Adenine, Guanine.
- The pyrimidine Cytosine is present in DNA & RNA.
- Thymine is seen in DNA and Uracil is seen in RNA.

Minor bases found in Nucleic acid:

➢ 5-methyl Cytosin – DNA.
➢ Hydroxymethylcytosin – present in Bacteria.
➢ Mono and di-N- methylated
➢ Adenine and Guanine - both are present in mamalian RNA.
➢ Pseudo Uridine – present in tRNA.

Free Nucleotides: (Biological important bases) The bases of hypoxanthine, xanthine, uric acid. The formed two are the intermediates in purine synthesis while uric acid is the end product of purine degradation.

Functions of Nucleotides:

1. Components of Nucleic acid: Nucleotides form the main component of nucleic acid. (Building blocks of nucleic acids – DNA, RNA).
2. Genetic material: DNA functions as the genetic material and transmits hereditary characters from parents to next generation.
3. Source of high energy: Nucleotides functions as the source of high energy Eg: ATP, UTP, and CTP.
4. CTP is required for synthesis of phosphoglycerides and sphingomyelin
5. Oxidative phosphorylation: ATP is involved in oxidative phosphorylation.
6. They regulate enzyme activity through feedback inhibition and allosteric regulation.
7. Co-enzyme: Certain nucleotides function as coenzymes Eg: UDP-glucouronic acid, CoA, FMN, and FAD.
8. UDP-Glucose is involved in glycogen synthesis.
9. UDP- glucuronic acid is involved in conjugation reactions eg: bilirubin.
10. Vitamins: Certain nucleotides function as vitamin B Eg: FMN, FAD, NAD.

11. They act as second messenger in mechanism of hormones action (cyclic AMP and cyclic GMP).

12. Synthetic nucleotides are used for the treatment of cancer (cytarabine, 5flouro or iodouracil, azauridine, azacytidine, azaguanine, mercaptopurineanddeoxyuridine which are incorporated in the DNA and inhibits cell division), hyperuricemia (allopurinol, a purine analog that inhibits purine synthesis by inhibiting the enzyme xanthine oxidase) and azathioprine is used during organ transplantation to inhibit rejection. Azathioprine is metabolized in the body to mercaptopurine.

Classification of nucleotides:

1. Adenosine nucleotides Ex: ATP, ADP, AMP, cyclic AMP
2. Guanosine nucleotides Ex: GTP, GDP, GMP, Cyclic GMP
3. Cytidine nucleotides Ex: CTP, CDP, CMP, CDP-choline
4. Uridine nucleotides Ex: UTP, UDP, UMP, UDP – glucose

Purine bases of plants: Plants contain certain methylated purines which are of pharmacological interest with varied applications.

1. Caffeine of coffee -- 1,3,7 – trimethyl xanthine
2. Theobromine of cocoa -- 3,7 – dimethyl xanthine
3. Theophylline of tea - 1, 7 – dimethyl xanthine

ATP: (Adenosine triphosphate) It is cellular energy currency The terminal two phosphates of ATP are high-energy phosphates. It forms most abundant free nucleotide in mammalian cells. Intra cellular concentration ranges about 1 mmol/L.

A large quantity of free energy is liberated due to the breakdown of these high energy phosphates like ATP to ADP+ P drives five important endergonic processes in the body which include.

➤ Muscular contraction.
➤ Nervous excitation (transmission of nerve impulses).
➤ Active transport
➤ Synthesis of important substances.
➤ Activation of metabolites.

cAMP: (Cyclic adenosine 3',5'- monophosphates)
The cAMP is formed from ATP by the action adenylyl cylclase enzyme and destroyed by phosphodiesterase. It bears cyclic structure. Its concentration is 1 nmol/L.
The cAMP is an important acts as a second messenger. Many hormones act through the formation or destruction of cAMP. The action of hormone depends on the concentration of cAMP in the target cells.

Adenosine 3'-phosphate -5'-phospho sulfate (PAPS)

- It contains Active sulfate to abbreviated as phosphoadenosine phosphosulfate donor for formation of sulfated proteoglycans, urinary metabolism of drugs are excreted as sulfate conjugates

Figure 1.4 Adenine Nucleotides

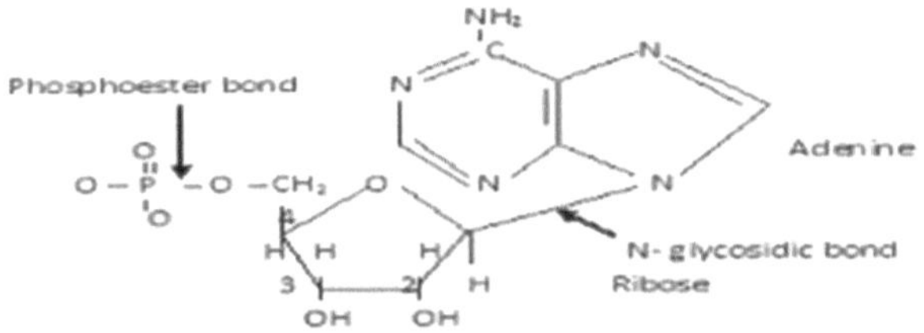

Adenosine Mono Phosphate (AMP)

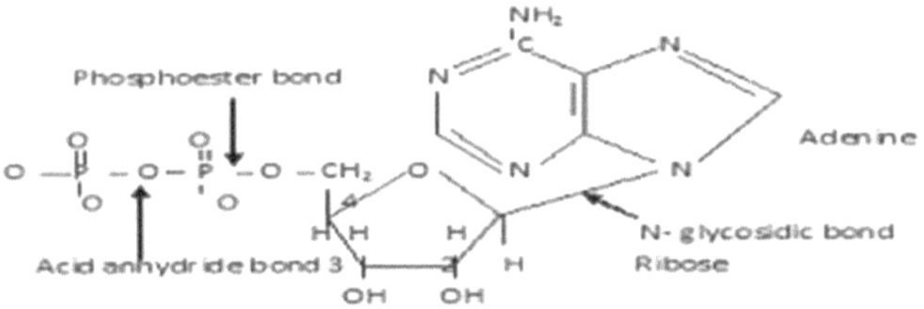

Adenosine Di Phosphate (ADP)

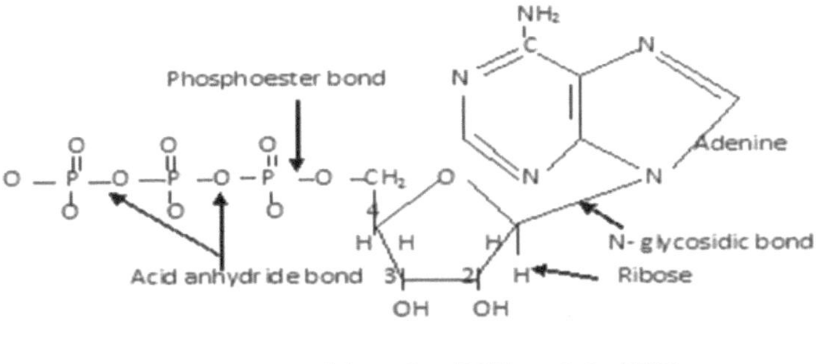

Adenosine Tri Phosphate (ATP)

Nucleotides:

Nucleotides are defined as phosphoric acid esters of nucleosides.

A Nucleotide is made up of three components namely or nitrogen base, pentose sugar and a phosphoric acid.

NUCLEOSIDES

Compounds that contain nitrogen bases and to pentose sugars from nucleosides. The pentose sugars are of two types, namely ribose sugar and deoxyribose sugar. Accordingly the nucleosides are broadly classified into two types, namely ribonucleosides and deoxyribonucleaside.

Figure 1.5 Deoxy Ribose sugar   **Figure 1.6 Ribose sugar**

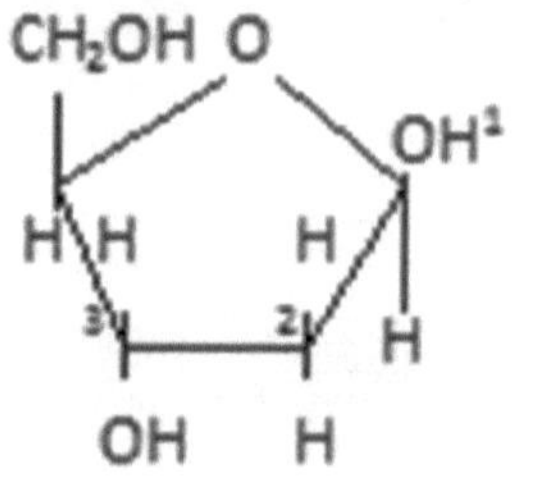

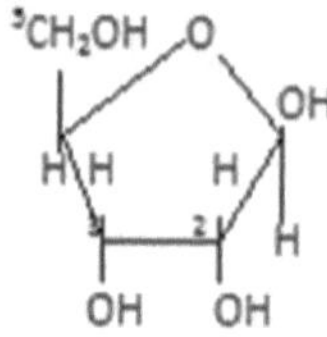

Ribose (Note: OH present in 2nd position)

The nitrogen bases are of two types, namely purines and pyrimidines. The purines are adenine and guanine. The pyrimidines are thymine, cytosine and Uracil.

The nucleosides are named according to the nature of nitrogen bases. Depending on nitrogen bases five types of nucleosides occur.

Synthetic analogs of purine/ pyrimidine nucleotides Mechanism Of action:

- Inhibition of specific enzymes which play a key role for nucleic acid synthesis.
- Incorporation of metabolites of the drug into nucleic acids that affect base pairing, hereditary transfer of information.

SYNTHETIC ANALOGS OF NUCLEOTIDE

- ➤ Inhibition of specific enzymes essential for nucleic acid synthesis.
- ➤ Incorporation of metabolites of the drug into nucleic acids that affect base pairing, essential for accurate transfer of information.
- ➤ It is possible to alter ring structure sugar moiety, and produce synthetic analongs of purines, pyrimidines, nucleside and useful in clinical medicine.

8

> ➤ Chemotherapeutic agents for cancer, AIDS and suppressors of immune rejection involved in organ transplantation.

1) **Allopurinal**---- these analogs are used for treatment of hyperuriemia, Gout. inhibits xanthine oxidase, 5- Fluorouracil, 6 – mercaptourine, 5 or 6- azocytisine (these are used for cancer as they inhibit proliferation) and 6 – azouridine, 8 – azoguanine.

1. **Azothiprine** ---- immunological rejection.
2. **Arabinosyladenine** ------ neurological disease viral encephalitis.
3. **Azotothymidine** and **Zidoverdine**----- HIV.
4. **Aravinosylcytosine** ----- used for cancer therapy as it interferes with DNA replication.
5. **Cytarabine** used in cancer and viral infections.
6. **Azathiopurine** used in organ transplantation
7. **5- iodo – deoxyuridine** used in herpetic keratitis

Table 1.1 Important Bases of nucleosides and nucleotides

S.No	Base	Ribonucleoside	Ribonucleotide 5'- monophosphate	Abbreviation
	Adenine	Adenosine	Adenosine 5'- monophosphate (or) adenylate	AMP
	Guanine	Guanosine	Guanosine 5' –monophosphate (or) Guanylate	GMP
	Cytosine	Cytidine	Cytidine 5' – monophosphate (or) cytidinate	CMP
	Uracil	Uridine	Uridine 5' – monophosphate (or) Uridylate	UMP

S.No	Base	Deoxyribonucleoside	Deoxyribonucleotide 5'- monophosphate	Abbreviation
	Adenine	Deoxyadenosine	DeoxyAdenosine 5'- monophosphate (or) Deoxyadenylate	dAMP

Guanine	Deoxyguanosine	DeoxyGuanosine 5' –monophosphate (or) DeoxyGuanylate	dGMP
Cytosine	Deoxycytidine	DeoxyCytidine 5' – monophosphate (or) Deoxycytidinate	dCMP
Thymine	Deoxythymine	Deoxythymine 5' – monophosphate(or) Deoxythymilate	dTMP

Chapter 2
DNA STRUCTURE AND FUNCTION

DNA is the chemical basis of hereditary and it forms the genetic material. It was discovered by Watson, Crick and Wilkins in early 1950s. It contains two polynucleotide strands, which are anti parallel; one running from 5` prime to 3`prime and the other is vice versa. The 5` prime of one strand is bound to the 3`prime of the other strand. DNA is built up of deoxy nucleotides which contains sugar deoxyribose. Each polynucleotide is made up of many small units called nucleotides. The nucleotides composed nitrogen bases, deoxyribose sugar and phosphoric acid. Each DNA is a polymer of about 10^{10} deoxyribonucleotides.

There are four different types of deoxyribo – nucleotides

1. deoxyadenylate (dAMP)
2. deoxythymidylate (dTMP)
3. deoxyguanidylate (dGMP)
4. deoxycytidylate (dCMP).

The back bone of the primary structure is the linear strand of interconnected sugar phosphate while the purine or pyrimidine protect from sugar residue. The sequence of the nucleotides on the DNA molecule forms the genetic information. The major function of the DNA is the transfer of genetic information from parents to offspring. The DNA is also controls regulation of all the cellular functions through regulation of gene expression (DNA, RNA and protein synthesis).

The Story of DNA discovery by Watson and Crick
DNA has a double helical structure formed by the two strands around a central axis. This model was proposed by Watson and crick. James Dewey Watson (born in 1928 at Chicago, USA) & Francis Harry Compton Crick (born in 1916 at Northampton, USA) James Watson was a child prodigy who was a student of University of Chicago at the age of 15. He graduated 1 in 1947 and obtained his

PhD from the University of Indiana in 1950. His excellency was with fellowship to study in Copenhagen but after a year there he moved to the Cavendish Laboratory, Cambridge, with the specific objective of studying the gene. There he met Francis Crick, who was working on protein structure for his PhD after starting as a physicist but becoming diverted to biology after the War. The famous fusion of great led Watson and Crick to deduce that DNA is a double helix has been described many times, notably by Watson in The Double Helix. The two shared the 1962 Nobel Prize with Maurice Wilkins.

The molecular details of DNA continue to unfold of a statement once quoted by the great Albert Einstein (Nobel laureate in Physics 1921) which means for every mile stone reached there is a sign post pointing to yet another. After the double helix, Watson and Crick moved in different paths. Watson returned to the USA in 1953 and eventually took up a professorship at Harvard University before moving in 1976 to the Cold Spring Harbor Laboratory on Long Island, where he became Director.

His research continued in fields like RNA synthesis, protein synthesis and role of viruses in cancer. He can also credited prime motivators behind the Human Genome Project, the ambitious research programmer whose goal was to unravel the complete nucleotide sequence of the human genome.

Crick stayed in Cambridge until moving to the Salk Institute in Southern California in 1977. During the 1950s and 1960s he played a key role in molecular biology and many of the great advances in understanding genes and gene expression aspects. His autobiography is What Mad Pursuit, Weidenfield and Nicolson, London 1989. Crick named his house at Cambridge the 'Golden Helix'. He had hung on the wall behind his desk in the Cavendish Lab the following motto: "Reading Rots the Mind."

Figure 2.1 Double helix structure of DNA

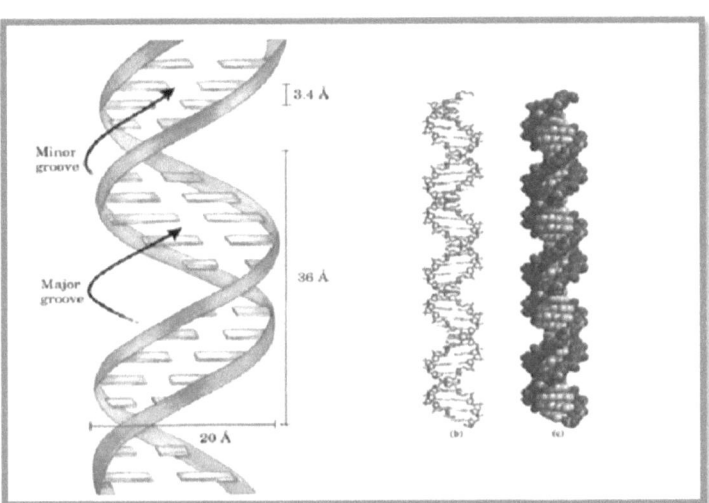

He often says:

"It is very difficult to explain something scientifically when you cannot explain what it is."

The two strands run antiparallel. Thus the polarity of two strands will be 3' – 5linear strand of interconnected sugar phosphate back bone with purine or pyrimidine forming ladder like structure projecting from the back bone. The two strands will be 3' – 5' strand called coding strand. The 5' – 3' strand called as non-coding strand or template strand. The two strands are bonded by hydrogen bonds – A = T by two bonds and G Ξ C by three bonds.

The phosphate and deoxyribose units are found on the periphery of the helix, forming backbone of ladder whereas the purine and pyrimidine bases occur in the centre of ladder, The planes of the bases are perpendicular to the helix axis. The planes of the sugars and bases are right angled. The diameter of the helix are 20 A°. The bases are 3. 4 A° apart along the helix axis and are related by a rotation of 36°. Therefore, the helical structure repeats after 10 residues on each chain i.e., at intervals of 34 Å. In other words, each turn of the helix contains 10 nucleotide residues.

The two chains are held together by hydrogen bonds between pairs of bases. Adenine always pairs with thymine through 2 hydrogen bonds and guanine similarly with cytosine with 3 hydrogen bonds. Thus making the two strands complementary. The individual hydrogen bonds are weak in nature but, as in the case of proteins, numerous bonds involved in the DNA molecule confer stability to it. It is now thought that the stability of the DNA molecule is primarily a consequence of van der Waals forces between the planes of stacked bases. The sequence of bases along a polynucleotide chain is not restricted in any way. The precise sequence of bases holds the genetic information.

As a corollary, the entire structure of a DNA Molecule resembles a winding staircase, with the sugar and phosphate molecules of the nucleotides forming the railings and the linked nitrogen base pairs (A – T and G – C) forming the staircase.

Figure 2.2 DNA structure

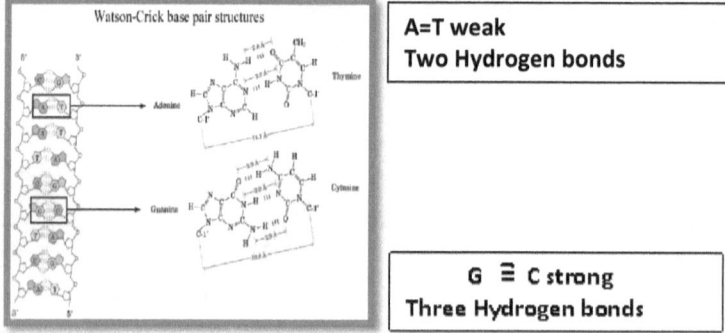

Chargaff's rule (it is molar equivalence between the purine and pyrimidine in DNA structure)

In one turn of double helix, 10 base pairs are present.

The pairing of bases is complementary to each other E.g., adenine is complementary to thymine Watson – Crick model of DNA helix.

Complimentarily is a term introduced into quantum theory by a physicist Niels Bohr (LT, 1885 – 1962), implying that evidence from atomic systems, that was obtained under different experimental conditions, cannot necessarily be comprehended by one single model. Thus, for example, the wave model of the electron is complementary to the particle model.

TYPES OF DNA

DNA is classified in various ways. First of all on depending the number of strands are present DNA is classified into several types. namely

1. Single strand DNA.
2. Double stranded DNA.

3. Triple stranded DNA.
4. Four- stranded DNA.

1. **Single strand DNA:** DNA of some viruses such as ϕ x 174 which attacks E.coli is single stranded.
    Depending on number of nucleotide residues, DNA is classified into 3 types
    A. A – DNA, B. B – DNA and C. Z- DNA
    a. A-DNA: It is double helical DNA having 11 residues perturn. Which is right handed helix. It is formed by the dehydration of B-DNA.
    b. B-DNA: This is the Watson and Crick double helix having 10 residues per turn. Which is also right handed. It is most common form.
    c. Z- DNA: It is a left handed double helix having 12 residues per turn and it forms zigzag model

Table 2.1 Differences between B-DNA and Z-DNA

S.NO:	B – DNA	Z –DNA
1	Right handed helical sense	Left handed helical sense
2	B-DNA is phosphate backbone is regular	The phosphate backbone of Z-DNA follows a zigzag course
3	B-DNA have same orientation	The adjacent sugar residues have opposite orientation
4	The angle of twist (rotation) per repeating unit 36^0 of mononucleotide in B-DNA	The angle of twist (rotation)per repeating unit (dinucleotide) in Z-DNA is 60^0
5	B-DNA one complete helix has only 10 base pairs or 10 repeating units	Z-DNA, one complete helix (i.e., a twist through 360^0) has 12 base pairs or 6 repeating dinucleotide units
6	B-DNA it is 34 A^0 long	In Z-DNA, one complete turn of helix is 45 A^0 long

Depending on the shape, DNA is classified into three types namely
Circular DNA
Relaxed DNA
Supercoiled DNA
Considering nucleotide sequence in the duplex DNA as the criteria there are two types

1. Palindromic DNA
2. Repetitive DNA or satellite DNA.

2. **Double stranded DNA:**
   This is otherwise known as double helical DNA in most of the organisms except a few viruses; the DNA is mostly a double stranded structure.

3. **Triple stranded DNA:** Triple –stranded DNA formation may occur due to additional strand and can selectively form two Hoogsteen hydrogen bonds to the adenine of A-T pair to form T-A-T purine, C-G-C pyrimidine.
   Triple – helical structure is less stable compared to double helix. Due to the fact that the three negatively charged backbone strands in triple helix results in an increased electrostatic repulsion.

4. Four-stranded DNA: Polynucleotides with very high contents of guanine can form a novel tetramer structure called Guanine quarters.
   Anti-parallel four strand DNA structure, referred to as G-tetra lexes.

Properties of DNA

The strands of double helix can separate or unwind during processes such as DNA replication. RNA transcription and genetic recombination. High temperature cause the complete unwinding of DNA. It is called as denaturation due to these hydrogen bonds between bases break and base pairs separate.

The temperature at which DNA is half denatured is called as melting temperature (Tm) of DNA. DNA rich in G-C pairs has a higher Tm than A-T pairs. Usually it is about 70^0 c. Reversal of denaturation is possible by slow cooling and the process is called renaturation as annealing.

Denaturation involves the following changes:

1. Increase in absorption of ultraviolet light (=Hyper chromic effect). As a result of resonance, all of the bases in nucleic acids absorb ultraviolet light. And all nucleic acids are characterized by a maximum absorption of UV light at wavelengths near 260 nm. In native DNA (base pairs are stacked) but denaturation, there occurs a marked increase in optical absorbency of UV light by pyrimidine and purine bases, an effect called hyperchromicity or hyperchromism which is due to unstacking of the base pairs. This change reflects a decrease in hydrogen-bonding. Hyperchromicity is observed not only with DNA but with other nucleic acids and with many synthetic polynucleotides which also possess a hydrogen-bonded structure.

2. Decrease in specific optical rotation. Native DNA exhibits a strong positive rotation which is highly decreased upon denaturation. This change is analogous to the change in rotation observed when the proteins are denatured.

3. Decrease in viscosity. The solutions of native DNA possess a high viscosity because of the relatively rigid double helical structure and long, rod like character of DNA. Disruption of the hydrogen bonds results in decreased in viscosity.

Effect of pH on denaturation

Denaturation of DNA helix also occurs at acidic and alkaline pH values at which ionic changes of the substituent's on the purine and pyrimidine bases can occur. In acid solutions near pH 2 to 3, at which amino groups bind protons, the DNA helix is disrupted. Similarly, in alkaline solutions near pH 12, the enolic hydroxyl groups ionize, thus preventing the keto-amino group hydrogen bonding.

Effect of temperature on denaturation:

The DNA double helix, although stabilized by hydrogen bonding, can be denatured by denaturing agents of which temperature is one agent. The temperature called denaturation temperature or melting because it occurs abruptly at a certain characteristics temperature called denaturation temperature or melting temperature Tm.

Nucleation reaction: In these hydrogen bonds between two complementary single strands; are formed which is a bimolecular, second-order reaction.

1. Zippering reaction: In this hydrogen bonds are formed between all the bases in the complementary strands; which is a unimolecular, first-order reaction
   The nature of melting transition is affected by
2. The (G + C) content of DNA: Higher the G+C content of DNA more stable will be the molecule and therefore higher will be its melting temperature compared to A+T content.
3. The nature of solvent: In low concentration of counter ion, denaturation occurs at relatively low temperatures and over a broad range, while at high concentration of counter ion, The Tm is raised and the transition is sharp.
4. The nature of DNA: Most DNA have varying G+C and A+T regions occurring as mosaics, which results in the two strands being held together at G+C regions. This region thus allows the reannealing of the broken H-bond, on lowering the temperature.

Molecular weight of DNA

DNA molecules are among the largest known. It is difficult to isolate DNA without fragmentation. The entire DNA of bacteria such as Escherichia coli has a molecular weight of 2.6×10^9. Viral DNAs range in size from about 1 to 350 x

10^6. The residue weight of a single nucleotide is 300 to 350. Thus, there are about 3,000 nucleotides per million molecular weight of DNA.

Along with this, the transition is accompanied by a change in intensity of the DNA where the single stranded molecule is denser than the corresponding duplex.

Renaturation of DNA: When 2 DNA strands are returned from the extreme conditions they may reassociate to re-form a double helix. Simple DNA molecules reanneal correctly and instantaneously than complex DNAs, by aligning perfectly. It at 4^0 it limits diffusion and prevents the separation of any DNA strand which have mismatched producing solutions of denatured DNA in case of complex molecules. The complexity of a DNA sample refers to time taken for DNA of given concentration to reanneal. The reassociation can be followed spectroscopically or by taking advantages of t he fact that a duplex DNA binds more strongly to hydroxyl apatite than a single stranded DNA. Another method makes use of S_1 nuclease an enzyme that preferentially digests single stranded DNA.

Buoyant Density of DNA: The percentage of G+C and A+T also influences the buoyant density of DNA in concentrated CsCl solutions G + C rich DNA has a higher buoyant density than A + T rich DNA.

Isolation and Separation of DNA: Phenol extraction is used widely method for the isolation of both DNA and RNA< which are retained in the aqueous phase while the denatured protein can be collected at the interface between this and the phenol phase which contains the lipids. RNA can be removed from the DNA by depending using pure pancreatic ribonuclease or by isopycnic ultracentrifugation in a gradient of CsCl. A density gradient established utilizing the buoyant densities of the molecules to be separated. Since equilibrium is established, in the process is also sometimes known as equilibrium ultracentrifugation. The buoyant density of double – stranded DNA varies with the G + C content, however RNA with high G+C content has a much higher buoyant density f (about 1.9 g/m) than double stranded DNA (about 1.7 g/m) which is in turn higher than of protein (about 1.3 g/m) Among all single stranded DNA has a slightly higher buoyant density.

Separation of bacterial plasmids from chromosome DNA uses the isopycnic ultracentrifugation. Chromosomal DNA is linear while plasmids are circular. The difference is exploited by addition of saturating concentration of intercalating fluorescent dye, ethidium bromide, where intercalation requires that the DNA strands be forced apart with a concomitant decrease in buoyant density and partial unwinding of the double helix. The unwinding of the double helix is hindered in the closed – circular plasmid molecule with the result that they bind less ethidium bromide and have a higher buoyant density than linear chromosome.

Chemical Reactions:
Some of the important reactions of the DNA are

(a) Strong mineral acids lead to depurination of Nucleic acid which lead to the conversion of sugars into furfural derivatives which give specific color reactions with orcinol (RNA) or diphenylamine (DNA).

(b) Nitrous acid reacts with amino groups to converting amino group to them into hydroxyls. Thus converting Cytosine → Uracil
Adenine → hypoxanthine
Guanine → Xanthine

Eukaryotic DNA:
Eukaryotic DNA is present in a relatively small number of chromosomes. No direct correlation can be established between the amount of DNA in the nucleus and the number of chromosomes in which it is contained. Somatic cells contain diploid number of chromosomes. The characteristic number and morphology of the chromosomes in a particular cell forms the Karyotype of that cell.

Table 2.2 DNA content and chromosome number

Organism	Haploid DNA	Content	Haploid chromosome
	Pico grams	Base pairs	Number
Simian Virus 40	0.000006	5.3×10^3	1
Herpes simplex	0.00017	151×10^3	1
E. coli	0.005	4.5×10^6	1
Drosophila melanogaster	0.17	0.15×10^9	4
Homo sapiens	2.7	2.4×10^9	23
Xenopuslaevis (Toad)	4.2	3.8×10^9	38
TriturusCristatus (newt)	35	31.5×10^9	12

The amount of DNA refers to an order of magnitude in excess is that required for the known gene coding capacities of the cells when the bulk of the DNA is not expressed.

The minimum size of genome i.e. amount of DNA per cell (C-value) is always in pace with the stage of evolutionary development. Certain amphibians have a 'C' value more than man other amphibian the reason being not clear. This phenomenon is known as the C value and paradox the species with greater amount of DNA would have the advantage of greater cording potential and the disadvantage here is the requirement to replicate very large amounts of DNA prior to cell division. Eukaryote DNA is divided into three frequency classes namely Unique DNA, moderately repetitive DNA and highly repeated DNA with a considerable overlap between the three categories.

Unique DNA

It comprises about half of the total haploid DNA content and consists of the Sequences coding for most enzyme functions for which there is only one or a small number of genes per haploid genome. In contrast to the prokaryotic genes which occupy a single uninterrupted sequence of DNA< the majority of Eukaryotic structural genes have extra sequences inserted into the middle of the gene. These intervening sequences are called introns, which may be small and single in some case like the case of the gene for tyrosine suppressor tRNA and large or multiple. In other cases these intervening regions are transcribed into RNA and then removed in the nucleus to produce the final mRNA. Such intervening sequences are less frequent in the lower Eukaryotes. Majority of structural genes display this phenomenon, and is not universal. The significance of introns is not properly understood and has been suggested to reflect the continual process of evolution within the Eukaryotic chromosome. Repetitive DNA includes all the rest of the DNA. The sequences represented in this group are generally thought to be those coding for proteins which form major structural components of the cell, eg. genes for rRNA, tRNA, histones etc.

Satellite DNA: It represents highly repeated sequences where a million or more copies per haploid genome which are usually quite short and are arranged in tandem arrays. The name is based on method of its isolation on CsCl buoyant density gradient of sheared DNA, where a satellite band is separated from the main DNA band due to their differing content of A & T residues. The distribution of satellite DNA among chromosomes varies some chromosomes have virtually no satellite while other (especially **y** chromosome) are largely composed of satellite sequences. Satellite DNA concentrated near the centromere of the chromosome in the hetero chromati9n fraction. The **function** of satellite which is not known properly. There occurs a contradictory idea regarding the transcription of satellite DNA and Its transcriptional inactivity lies within its localization in heterochromatin.

Interspersed Repetitive DNA: It differs from the satellite DNA by having sequences dispersed singly throughout the genome. They are of two classes.

  (a) Short interspersed nuclear elements (SINES) consisting of repeats shorter than 500 bp and the long interspersed nuclear elements (LINES).

Example of SINES is the Alu family in human cells (it derives its name from the presence of a single site for the restriction enzyme Alu I in the repeat). The Alu sequence is transcribed and it is believed to have become dispersed throughout the genome by reverse transcription and reintegration therefore it is termed as Retroposon.

Fold back DNA or Palindromic DNA these sequences comprise 3 – 6% of Eukaryotic DNA. The size range is from 300 to 1200 bp.

5' TGCGATGC: CGATCGCA 3'
3' ACGCTACG: CGTACGCT 5'

Genes

Genes are the basic physical & functional units of heredity. A gene is a specific sequence of nucleotide bases, which is carry the information required for constructing proteins, which provide the structural components of cells and tissues as well as enzymes for essential biochemical reactions. The human genome is estimated to comprise at least 100,000 genes. Human genes vary widely in numerous aspects like length, often extending over thousands of bases, but only about 10% of the genome is known to include the protein-coding sequences (exons) of genes. Interspersed within many genes are intron sequences, which have no coding function. The balance of the genome is maintained in the forms of other non coding regions (such as control sequences and intragenic regions), whose functions are obscure. All living organisms are composed largely of proteins; humans can synthesize at least 100,000 different kinds. Proteins are large, complex molecules made up of subunits called amino acids. Twenty different kinds of amino acids are usually found in proteins. Within the gene, each specific sequence of three DNA bases (codons) directs the cell's protein-synthesizing machinery to add specific amino acids. For example, the base sequence ATG codes for the amino acid methionine. A codon which includes 3 bases code for1 amino acid, the protein coded by an average-sized gene (3000 bp) will contain 1000amino acids. The genetic code is thus a series of codons that specify the sequence of aminoacids required to make up specific proteins. The protein-coding instructions from the genes are transmitted indirectly through messenger ribonucleic acid (mRNA), a transient intermediary molecule similar to a single strand of DNA. For the information within a gene to be expressed, a complementary RNA strand is produced (a process called transcription) from the DNA template in the nucleus.

Chromosome

The 24 in number and they are physically distinct Microscopic units called chromosomes. 2 sets of chromosomes, 1 set obtained from given by each parent. Each set has 23 single chromosomes—22 of which autosomes and an X or Y sex Chromosome. (A normal female is represented by pair of X chromosomes and a male represented by X and Y pair.)

Chromatin Structure

In the interphase the chromosome is referred to as chromatin. They are subdivided into two classes – Euchromatin and Heterochromatin. Heterochromatin comprises the dense readily stained areas of the nucleus or chromosome and was thought to represent inactive chromatin. The Euchromatin is more loosely packed, which was thought to represent the transcriptionally active material.

Chromatin consists of DNA, RNA and proteins. In general the amount of protein is equal to or greater than the amount of DNA while the amount of RNA is comparatively small.

The protein content of chromatin can be further subdivided into histone and non-histone proteins.

Histone

The histones are basic proteins of low molecular weight. Each molecule consists of a hydrophobic core region with one or two basic arms. They are classified into five types namely H_1, H_2A, H_2B, H_3 and H_4.

H_1 is lysine-rich protein consisting of about 216 amino acids in which sequence is highly conservation among eukaryotes particularly at the central a Polar Regions. H_2A and H_2B are even more highly conserved and are forms lysine rich histones. The most conserved of all are the Arg-rich histones H_3 and H_4.

The effect of variation in sequence of histones on chromatin structure is not clear. However the histones may be methylated, phosphorylated, etc. and which has an affect on the interaction of histones with each other or with the DNA.

In sperm cells histone are replaced by other small basic proteins known as protamine.

In the absence of DNA the **'core'** histones associate with each other, the predominant species being a homotypic tetramer in the case of H_3 and H_4 a dimer in case of H_2A, H_2B.

Non Histone Proteins

They occur in approximately equal amounts to histones. Some have an enzymatic role involved in replication and transcription, other resembles the histone being of low mol. Wt. are known as high mobility group of HMG proteins. They are also basic like the histones and play a structural role, but differ from histones in being only loosely associated with chromatin.

Nucleosome

The DNA of human cell is ranges about 1m in length and is condensed in a cell nucleus whose diameter is of the order of 10 μm. Thus is packing within the nucleus accessibility during replication. Histones and some other chromosomal proteins form the complex of DNA – histone forms the beads called nucleosomes in which the double-stranded DNA forms the string.

Each nucleosome is composed of two molecules each of histones, H_2A, H_2B, H_3 and H_4 and about 200 bp of DNA. The H_2A, H_2B, H_3 and H_4 molecules form a protein complex called the histone octamer and DNA is wrapped around the octomer. About, 146 bp of DNA are in close contact with the histone octamer to form a nucleosome core particle. The DNA to the linker DNA and to the nucleosome core particle. H_1 is responsible for higher order chromatin structures. The DNA is thus not only compacted in chromatin it is also rendered partially resistant to nuclease action.

Higher levels of Chromatin Structure:

The packaging of DNA into nucleosome results in 10 fold reduction in chromosome chain length and this reduces even further upon higher levels of DNA packaging. The beads on a string structure are itself coiled into a solenoid to yield the 30 mm fiber. The adjacent molecules of H_1 bind cooperatively in such a way that nucleosomes form compact and stable form of chromatin. This achieves a further fourfold reduction in the length.

The 30 nm fibers some times are attached to a non-histone protein scaffold that resolves the fibers in large loops. There occur 2000 such loops on a large chromosome. Such packaging results in chromosomes of 5 – 10 μm in length and 1 μm in diameter. The organization of the DNA into loops accounts for the remaining 200-fold condensation in the length of the DNA.

Extra Nuclear DNA (Mitochondrial DNA)

It is a cyclic, double stranded super coiled molecule with an exception of linear Mitochondrial DNA in paramecium.

Mammalian mitochondrial DNA are not packaged into nucleosomes. These are about 15 kbp long and can therefore code for 15 to 20 proteins. Yeasts have 75 k long base pairs, plant mitochondrial DNA are still longer.

Mitochondrial DNA codes only for a small proportion protein of mitochondrial yet it is described as a "lesson in Economy". Introns are absent in mammalian mitochondrial genes but present in some yeast genes. There are genes for rRNAs, tRNAs and some other proteins of the ETC present on the mitochondrial DNA.

The mitochondrial origin they rose as symbiotic prokaryotes providing oxidative metabolism to their pre Eukaryotic hosts. Throughout evolution, most of the genes were transferred from the symbiotic to the nuclear DNA of the host leaving behind only the remnants.

Chloroplast DNA

It is a little larger compared to mitochondrial DNA containing 150 kbp. There are many copies of the DNA within the chloroplast, unlike that seen in mitochondria. Which holds occur in essential membrane components, rRNA, tRNA. All the chloroplast DNA are cyclic and super coiled forms.

Bacterial DNA

Bacteria which possess the full complement of bacterial genes are referred to as wild type bacterial or prototroph and the mutants are classified on the basis of their missing function a nutritional mutant is referred to as an auxotroph. Most bacteria carry all their genetic information on single, circular chromosome which possess small extra chromosomal elements known as Plasmids which carry genes for drug resistances. Chromosome of E.coli for example, is a single cyclic duplex molecule of 4.5 million base pairs having an effective circumference of 1 mm which should be packed in the cell which is 1 μm and which requires a complex packaging is required. Achieved by two main mechanisms.

(a) First the DNA is folded into loop ranging between 40 and 100 loops.
(b) Each of these quasi circles is itself supercoiled independently of others.

Plasmids

They are duplex, super coiled stable DNA elements which exist in bacteria and some Eukaryotes. Larger ones are present in only one copy while the smaller may have more copies per cell say upto 20. Which autonomous and self replicating.

Chapter 3
RNA

RNA is a polymer of nucleotide of Adenine, Cytosine, Guanine, and Uracil. It is different from the DNA in having composed of one polynucleotide strand, which contains ribose instead of deoxyribose, sugar with nitrogenous bases are A, G, C and U. RNA is forms T is absent in RNA and the guanine content is not equal to cytosine like in DNA molecule. The second nucleic acid in nature. Nucleotides in RNA are joined together by 3'– 5' phosphodiester bonds and occur in nucleus, ribosomes, mitochondria and cytoplasm. The pentose sugar is D-ribose. RNA is single stranded. There is interchain hydrogen bonding between G-C and A-U thus conforming secondary and tertiary structure of RNA causing the folding of molecules into three dimensional structures. Some RNA in the form of ribosome acts as catalyst of reactions.

In RNA the purines and pyrimidines are not present in equal amount which indicates RNA does not follow Chargaff's rule).

TYPES OF RNA
There are mainly three types:

1. Messenger RNA (mRNA).
2. Transfer or soluble RNA (tRNA).
3. Ribosomal RNA (rRNA).

The main function of the RNA is protein synthesis in human cells but some small nuclear RNA (snRNA) exact which are not involved in protein biosynthesis which have some role in processing of RNA. A large processor of mRNA called as heterogeneous nuclear RNA (hnRNA) is also found in the nucleus.

1. **Messenger RNA (mRNA):** Messenger RNA is a nucleic acid which carries genetic information for protein synthesis from the DNA to the cytoplasm. The term mRNA was coined by JACOB and MONAD in 1961 mRNA

forms about 3 to 5% of total cellular RNA. It is formed with the help of DNA template strand during the process called as transcription. Catalysed by the enzyme RNA polymerase. It carries specific sequences of nucleotides in triplets called as codons. messenger RNA (mRNA) is copied from one strand of DNA and it transfers the genetic information from DNA to the protein synthesis machinery in the rough endoplasmic reticulum.

2. The released introns are known as microRNA and they are involved in cancer causation thus the research in this way is directed towards using the microRNA molecules as targets for cancer therapies.

3. mRNA is synthesized as premature molecule known as heterogenous nuclear RNA (hnRNA). The mature mRNA is composed of a sequence of nucleotides (Exons) capped at the 5` prime by 7-methyl guanosine Tri Phosphate and tailed at the 3` prime by poly Adenine. The Exons are composed of a triplet nucleotide sequence (codons) that serve as codes for amino acids.

4. It carries mainly A-G C-U as the major bases and methyl purines and hydroxyl methyl purines as minor bases. mRNA plays important role in protein biosynthesis. The 3' – OH end contains 3- 250 adenylate ribonucleotide residues forms poly-A tail (20-250 adenylate residues) which is essential for maintaining intracellular stability and preventing the attack of 3 exonucleases and 5' – OH end contains 7-methyl guanidylate residue called as cap end which is useful for preventing attack of exonucleases and increasing half life of mRNA.

Structure of mRNA: A – U, C-G phosphate group + ribose sugar.

mRNA coding for single polypeptide chain is called monocistronic and that coding for many polypeptide chains is called polycistronic mRNA. The mRNA is a single stranded polynucleotide chain containing 500 to 1500 nucleotides. The mRNA carries genetic information's from DNA. The genetic information carried by the mRNA is called genetic code. The genetic code is the sequence of nitrogen bases in mRNA. The genetic code is formed of several codons. Each codon is a sequence of three nitrogenous bases which codes for one aminoacid. As each codon is formed of three nitrogen bases, it is called a triplet code. Among RNAs, mRNA is the longest one. Most of the mRNA contains 900 to 15000 nucleotide. If the mRNA contains 900 nucleotides the polypeptide chain synthesized by this mRNA will contain 300 aminoacid.

Function of mRNA

The mRNA acts as a messenger. mRNA carries the genetic information in the form of triplet code from the DNA. The code on mRNA decides the type of protein to be synthesized.

Transfer or soluble RNA (tRNA)

- The tRNA is a ribonucleic acid which transfers the activated amino acids to the ribosomes site of protein synthesis. It is supernatant configuration also called soluble RNA or supernatant RNA present in cytoplasm. They are small single stranded polynucleotides. There are 20 specific tRNA for 20 Aas. tRNA is famous as the adaptor molecule because it translates.
- The tRNA has a clover leaf shape because of internal hydrogen bonding. It has five types of arms; the acceptor arm, anticodon arm, D arm, TΨC arm and extra arms. The D, TΨC and extra arms help to define specific tRNA. The function of the acceptor is accepting the amino acids depending on codon the amino acids bind an A moiety of a CCA sequence on the 3` prime of the acceptor arm. The anticodon arm is composed of a three nucleotide sequence and it is responsible for binding the codons on the mRNA.
- There are 61 tRNA molecules in each cell, responsible for carrying the 20 proteinic amino acids. i.e. one amino acid can be carried by more than one tRNA (degeneracy) while one tRNA carries only one amino acid (un ambiguity).
- Functions of tRNA include transferring of amino acids from the cytoplasm to the rough endoplasmic reticulum and translating the sequence of nucleotides (codons) on the mRNA into amino acid sequence (protein).

Structure of tRNA

The tRNA is made up of 75 to 95 nucleotide units called ribonucleotides.
A part from regular nucleotides some rare bases do occur like pseudouracil (ψ) and thymine are present.
Each single strand of tRNA molecule remained folded to form a cloverleaf secondary structure. It is stabilized by H-bonds.

All tRNA contain 5 arms or loops.

- **Acceptor arm**: This consists of unpaired sequence of C-C-A at 3' end also called as acceptor end. The 3' – OH of adenine binds the specific amino acids and assists in protein biosynthesis.
- **Anti codon arm**: It carries specific sequence of three bases constitutes the anticodon. It recognizes codon of the template mRNA and adds amino acids corresponding to recognized codons The interaction of codon of mRNA and anticodon of t-RNA takes place on the ribosomes. These anticodons have a crucial role in protein biosynthesis.
- **D- arm:** It contains base dihydrouridine (DHU). It is required for the proper recognition of a given rRNA by its charging enzyme amino acyl tRNA synthatase.
- **T-arm:** It contains thymine, pseuduridine and cytosine.
- **Variable arm:** It is extra arm and varies depending upon number bases in this arm ex class I tRNA – 3 to 5 bases and Class II t RNA – 13 to 21 bases.

Figure 3.1: Structure of tRNA

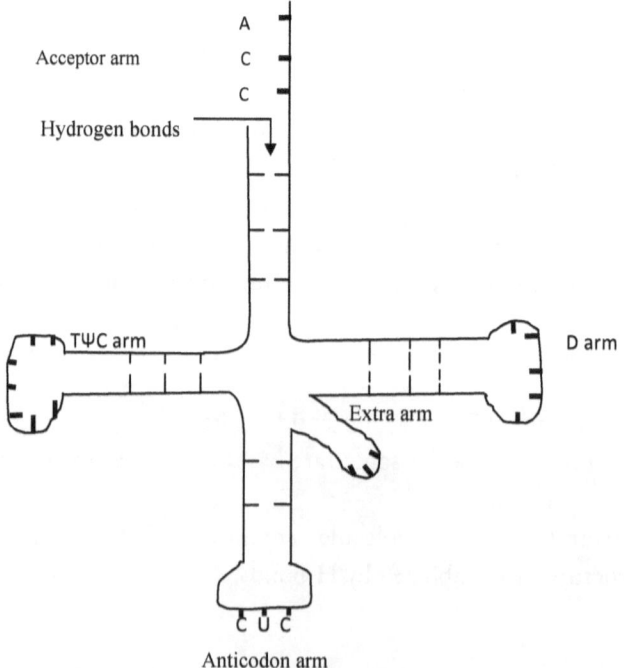

Acceptor arm
Hydrogen bonds
TΨC arm
D arm
Extra arm
Anticodon arm

5. RIBOSOMAL RNA (rRNA)

Ribosomal RNA is a ribonucleic acid present in the ribosomes and hence it is called ribosomal RNA. They constitute 80% of cellular RNA.

It is also called insoluble RNA. There are different types of rRNA depending on their sedimentation velocity coefficient which is measured by Svedberg unit (S). The Svedberg unit is controlled by the size and shape of molecules. The rRNA types include 5S, 5.8S,16S, 18S, 23S and 28S rRNA molecules. rRNA molecules are major components of ribosomes and the 23S and 28S act as an enzyme (peptidyletransferase) and minor components include 5S, 5.8S,16S, 18S Ribosomes are nuclear proteins composed of proteins and ribosomal RNA molecules. They are classified to **Eukaryotic** and **prokaryotic** ribosomes. The two are composed of two subunits; large and small subunits. Ribosomes are located on the rough endoplasmic reticulum and together they constitute the protein synthesizing machinery. The Eukaryotic ribosome is famous as the 80S ribosome containing 40S subunit and 60S subunit. The 40S (small unit) contains the 18S rRNA while the 60S (large subunit) contains the 5S, 5.8S and 28S rRNA molecules.

The small unit of the prokaryotic ribosome (70S ribosome)is known as the 30S and it contains the 16S ribosomal RNA. The 50S marks large unit of the prokaryotic ribosome and it contains the 5S and 23S ribosomal RNA molecules.

Types of rRNA

The rRNAs are classified into 7types according to their sedimentation co-efficient. They are following

28 s rRNA	23 s rRNA
18 s rRN A	16 s rRNA seen in prokaryotic cell
5.8 s rRNA	5 s rRNA seen in Eukaryotic cells

Of these 28 s rRNA is larger subunit and smaller subunits 18 s rRNA, 5.8 s rRNA, and 5 s rRNA are existing in eukaryotic cells. 23 s rRNA is larger subunit and smaller subunits 16 s rRNA, and 5 s rRNA are existing in prokaryotic cells. In eukaryotic ribosomes, the large 60 s ribosomal subunit contains 28 s rRNA, 5.8 s rRNA and 5 s rRNA. The small 40 s ribosomal sub unit contains 18 s rRNA. In prokaryotic 23 s rRNA and 5 s rRNA. The small 30 s ribosomal sub unit contains 16 s rRNA.

Functions of rRNA: Though the rRNA constitutes the bulk of the cytoplasmic RNA, its function is not clearly known. However it is believed that rRNA plays the major role in protein synthesis.

Table 3.1 DIFFERENCES BETWEEN DNA AND RNA

	DNA	RNA
Site	Mostly in nucleus	Mostly in cytoplasm
Function	Carries information for genetic transmission and protien synthesis	Synthesis of protein
Bases	Adenine, guanine, cytosine, thymine	Adenine, guanine, cytosine, Uracil
Sugar	Deoxyribose	Ribose
Structure	Double stranded	Single stranded
Purine/ pyrimidine contact	$A + G = T + C$ (almost equal)	$A + G \neq U + C$ (not equal)
Types	B-DNA, A-DNA, Z-DNA	m-RNA, tRNA, rRNA
Stability	Alkali stable	Alkali labile
Genetic material	It is a genetic material in all organisms	It is a genetic material in certain viruses
Component	It is a component of Chromosome	It is a component of Ribosome
Formation	It can replicate it self	It can't replicate itself. It is formed by DNA
Primer	A primer is needed for replication	No primer is need for transcription
Molecular Weight	It's M.W varies from 2 to 6 millions	It's M.W varies from 25,000 to 2 millions
Genetic information and Mutation	They carry genetic information from one generation of cells to the next and undergo mutation	They carry no genetic information and undergo no mutation

Structure	They contain 1,600 to 9000 nucleotides. The molecular long and thread. Like having a length of about 250 times greater than their breadth. Their structure is highly complex	They contain 60 to 6,000 nucleotides. The molecules are unbranched. The structure is less rigid
Strands	They have sense and antisense strands	The sequence of RNA molecule is the same as that of the antisense strand of DNA.

Chapter 4

PURINE RING STRUCTURE

PRPP:

- *PRPP is Phosphoribosyl pyrophosphate. It is synthesized from ribose-5 (P). which is It is required for the conversion of Nicotinate to Nicotinate Mono Nucleotide (NMN).*
- This forms the substrate for both denovo synthesis and also salvage pathways of both purine and pyrimidine synthesis.

Figure 4.1 Purine ring structure and source of individual molecules

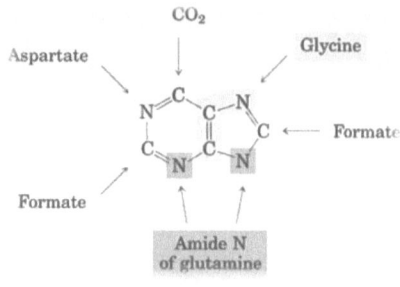

Formation of PRPP:

- It is formed by transfer of pyrophosphate from ATP to carbon 1 of α-D-ribose- 5-P, catalysed by **PRPP -synthase.**

MATERIALS REQUIRED: (Purine ring is built on ribose -5- phosphate)

- PRPP (5-phosphoribosyl-1-pyrophosphate)
- Enzymes: various synthases, transferases, carboxylases.
- Energy: ATP Uses 6 high energy phosphate bonds.
- Aminoacid and derivatives: glycine, aspartic acid, glutamine
- CO2: from HCO3
- Coenzymes /factors: formyl THF, Mg^{++}
- The structural analogs of folic acid (eg: methotrexate) are widely used to control cancer. They inhibit the synthesis of purine nucleotides and thus nucleic acids. These inhibitors also affect the proliferation of normally

growing cells. This causes many side-effects including anemia, baldness, scaly skin etc.

Addition of N9 – in purine synthesis:

- Amide group of glutamine is transferred to C1 of
- PRPP by **PRPP glutamyl amidotransferase, forming**
- 5-phosphoribosyl -1- amine. **It is rate limiting step**

Regulation of purine synthesis:

1. The committed step in denovo synthesis is **PRPP glutamyl amidotransferase**. Which is a regulating step regulated by AMP and GMP act as allosteric modifiers.
2. **PRPP synthatase** is important enzyme that regulates purine synthesis. Inhibited allosterically by feedback effects of PRPP, purine nucleotides AMP, GMP, ADP, GDP.

Salvage pathway of purines synthesis:

- In this pathway free purines (adenine, guanine & hypoxanthine) are formed in the normal turnover of nucleic acids & also obtained from the dietary sources.
- Through salvage pathway corresponding nucleotides are formed form purines catlysed by phosphoribosyl transferase and the formation of AMP from adenine.
- Similarly hypoxanthine-guanine phosphoribosyl transferase (HGPRT) converts guanine & hypoxanthine respectively, to GMP & IMP.
- Phosphoribosyl pyrophosphate (PRPP) is the donor of ribose 5 phosphate in the salvage pathway.

The salvage pathway is of great significance in certain tissues such as erythrocytes & brain where denovo synthesis of purine nucleotides is not operative.

In this pathway nucleotides are degraded resulting in recycling of purines.

1. The denovo synthesis is expensive.
2. does not occur in all tissues capable of denovo synthesis
   Eg: RBC, Brain, neutrophils.

They lack PRPP amidotransferase.

3. Nucleotides are but converted to nucleosides before entering cell membrane nucleosidases.
4. After entering into cell, nucleoside is converted again to nucleotide (by kinase)/ or degraded to corresponding base (by nucleoside phosphorylase)

Salvage pathway – It is two step synthesis recycling catalysed by enzyme and Nucleoside phosphorylase – nucleoside kinase. This pathway ensures Recycling of purines by degradation of nucleotides.

Lesch-Nyhan syndrome:

This disorder is due to the deficiency of hypoxanthine-guanine phosphoribosyltransferase (HGPRT), an enzyme of purine salvage pathway. Lesch-nyhan syndrome is a sex-linked metabolic disorder due to occurance structural gene for HGPRT on the X-chromosome. It is common among the males and is characterized by excessive uric acid production (often gouty arthritis). This is characterized by neurological abnormalities such as mental retardation, aggressive behavior, learning disability etc.

The patients suffering from this disorder have an irresistible urge to bite their fingers and lips, often causing self-mutilation. There is over production of uric acid in lesch-nyhan syndrome levels. HGPRT deficiency results in the accumulation of PRPP and depletes in GMP and IMP, ultimately leading to increased synthesis and degradation of purines. The biochemical bases for the neurological symptoms observed in Lesch-Nyhan syndrome are not clearly understood. This may be related to the dependence of brain on the salvage pathway for de novo synthesis of purine nucleotides. Uric acid is not toxic to the brain, since patients with severe hyperuricemia (not related to HGPRT deficiency) do not exhibit any neurological symptoms.

Inheritance pattern -- X-linked recessive
Defective enzyme is (salvage pathway) -- *hypoxanthine guanine phoshoribosyl transferase (HGPRT)*

Features:

- Only males are suffer, as structural gene for HGPRT is on X- chromosome and females act as carriers.
- Characterized by excess formation of uric acid.

- Nephrolithiasis
- Selfmutilation
- Neurological abnormalities like mental -retardation, aggressive behavior, learning disabilities occur.
- Neurological symptoms may be due to **dependence of brain** on the salvage pathway.

PRPP:

- *It refers to* **5- phoshoribosyl – 1- pyrophosphate.**
- This is **substrate for both purine and pyrimidine synthesis.**

Formation of PRPP: first step in purine synthesis

- It is formed by transfer of pyrophosphate from ATP to
- carbon 1 of α-D-ribose- 5-P, catalysed by **PRPP -synthase.**

Addition of N9 – in purine synthesis:

➤ Amide group of **glutamine** is transferred to C1 of
➤ PRPP by **PRPP glutamylamidotransferase, forming**
➤ 5-phosphoribosyl -1- amine. **It is rate limiting step of purine synthesis.**

Inhibitors of purine synthesis:

➤ 6-mercaptopurine: Inhibits conversion of adenylo succinate to AMP.
➤ Azaserine: Inhibits incorporation of N_3 in the purine ring from glutamine.

Purine Catabolism and its disorders:

- The end product of purine metabolism in humans is uric acid.

- The nucleotide monophosphates (AMP, IMP & GMP) nucleosidase enzyme converts to their respective nucleoside forms (adenosine, inosine & guanosine).

- Removal of the amino group, either from AMP or adenosine to produces IMP or inosine Xanthine oxidase is an important enzyme that converts hypoxanthine to xanthine, & xanthine to uric acid.

- This enzyme contains FAD, Molybdenum & Iron, & is exclusively found in liver & small intestine.

- Xanthine oxidase liberates H2O2 & H2O both which proved harmful to the tissues.

- Catalase cleaves H2O2 to H2O & O2.respectively.

- Uric acid (2,6,8-trioxopurine) is the final excretory product of purine metabolism in humans.

- Uric acid can serve as an important antioxidant by getting itself converted non enzymatically to allantoin.

- It is believed that the antioxidant role of ascorbic acid in primates is replaced by uric acid, since these animals have lost the ability to synthesize ascorbic acid.

Figure 4.2 Catabolism of Purines

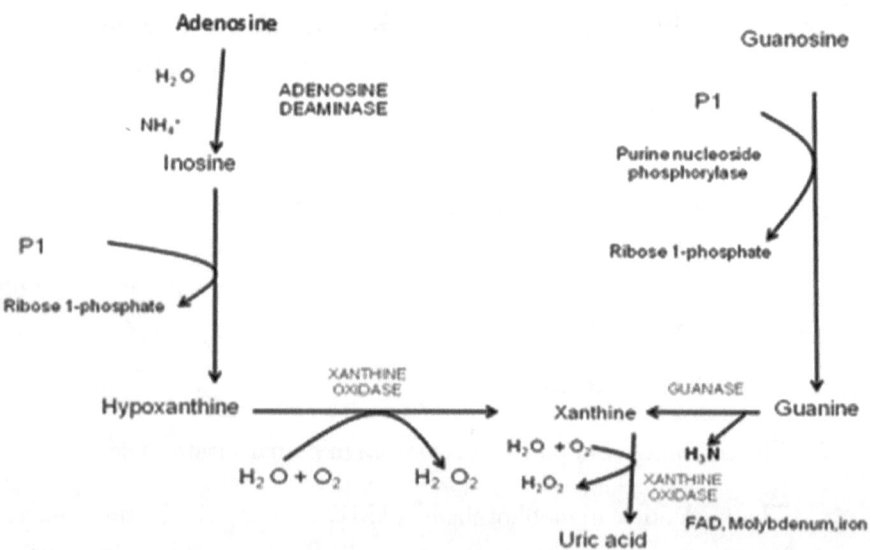

Above the picture shows Formation of uric acid from purine nucleosides involving purine bases hypoxanthine xanthine and guanine. Purine deoxyrinucleosides are degraded by the similar catabolic pathway and enzymes. Which exist in the mucosa of the mammalian gastrointestinal tract.

Purine Catabolism and its disorders:

- The end product of purine catabolism is uric acid in humans.
- Uric acid is degraded into allantoic acid and finally to ammonia in animals other than man.
- *Uric acid is 2, 6, 8 –trioxy purine.*

It acts as antioxidant by converting itself into allantoin.

Uric acid

- *Normal serum concentration*: **3 to 7 mg /dl** in males
  2 to 5 mg/dl in females
- *Miscible pool* – the quantity of uric acid present in body water.
  It is on average of 1130mg
- *Daily turnover*: 500 to 600 mg synthesized
  400 to 600 mg/day excreted
- Uric acid is **cleared** from the body by both glomerular **filtration** and tubular **secretion**.

Hyperuricemia and gout: Uric acid is the end product of purine metabolism in humans.

- Hyperuricemia refers to an elevation in the serum uric acid concentration.

- This is sometimes associated with increased uric acid excretion (Uricosuria)

- GOUT is metabolic disease associated with overproduction of uric acid. Metabolic changes in gout (Figure 4.3)

- At the physiological pH, uric acid occur in a more soluble form as sodium urate.

- In severe hyperuricemia, crystals of sodium urate get deposited in the soft tissues, particularly in the joints such deposits are Tophi.

- The normal concentration of uric acid in the serum of adults is in the range of 3-7 mg / dl. In women, it is slightly lower (by about 1 mg) than in men. The daily excretion of uric acid is about 500-700 mg.

- These deposits cause inflammation in the joints resulting in a painful gouty arthritis. Typical gouty arthritis affects first metatarsophalangeal joint. (GREAT TOE).

- Sodium urate &/or uric acid may also precipitate in kidneys & ureters that result in renal damage & stone formation.

- Historically, gout is a disorder related to high living, over-eating & alcohol consumption.

Formation of *5- phoshoribosyl – 1- pyrophosphate.*

Clinical features:

- Attacks are precipitated by alcohol intake.

- Often patient suffer few drinks, go to sound sleep symptomless, but are awakened during early hours by severe joint pains.

The prevalence of gout is about 3 / 1,000 persons, mostly affecting males. Deficiency leads to severe combined immunodeficiency disease [SCID], [Autosomal recessive]

Types of gout:

1. ***Primary gout:*** Metabolic Causes:
   - Variant form of PRPP synthetase- are not under allosteric regulation. (increased activity)
   - The defective enzyme - 5- phosphoribosyl- amidotransferase is active but inactive to feedback control.(increased activity)
   - Deficiency of enzyme of **salvage pathway –HGPRT** deficiency leading to **Lesch-Nyhan syndrome**.
2. **Secondary gout:**
   a) **Overproduction of uircacid – due to enhanced *turnover rate of nucleic acids***
      i) Increased tissue turn over due to **psoriasis.**
      ii) Rapidly growing malignant tissues-**leukemias.**
      iii) Increased tissue break down – **after treatment for large tumour masses.** (with radiation, chemotherapy)

b) **Reduced excretion of uric acid**
- Increased alcohol consumption results in accumulation of lactic acid leading to lactic -acidosis. Lactic acid inhibits uric acid excretion.
- Thiazide diuretics inhibit tubular secretion of uric acid.
- It results in Renal failure.

c) **OTHERS**
VONGIERKE'S DISEASE
Elevated glutathione reductase

Treatment:

- Low intake of purine diet
- Restriction of alcohol is important in treating Vangierke's disease.

Drugs:

1. **Uricosuric drugs** – probenecid, salicylates, halofenate
2. **Enzyme inhibitors – allopurinol**

Action of allopurinol:
Allopurinol $\rightarrow$ alloxanthine
      xanthine oxidase
        inhibits
Xanthine and hypoxanthine are more soluble and excreted easily.

Lesch-Nyhan syndrome:
Inheritance pattern -- X-**linked recessive**
Enzyme defect (salvage pathway) -- *hypoxanthine guanine phoshoribosyl transferase (HGPRT)*
    $\downarrow$
  Rate of salvage pathway decreases
    $\downarrow$
Accumulation of intracellular PRPP and decrease in GMP and IMP, the inhibitory nucleotides
    $\downarrow$
Increased production and degradation of purine nucleotides.

Features:

- Only males are suffers, as structural gene for HGPRT is on X- chromosome and females act as carriers.
- Characterized by excess formation of uric acid.
- Nephrolithiasis
- Selfmutilation
- Neurological abnormalities like mental -retardation, aggressive behavior, learning disabilities occur.
- Neurological symptoms may be due to **dependence of brain on purines,** fomed in the salvage pathways.

Adenosine deaminase deficiency and purine- nucleoside phosphorylase deficiency:

Both are inherited as ***autosomal recessive.***

In severe combined immunodeficiency disease there is decreased T cells, B cells and natural killer cells. Lymphocytes have the highest activity of this cytoplasmic enzyme. ADA deficiency leads to increased amount of adenosine. Both increased levels of adenosine and deoxyadenosine are toxic to the cells.

1. Adenosine is converted to ribonucleotides or deoxyribonucleotides by cellular kinases. As dATP level rises it inhibits the enzyme ribonucleotide reductase, thereby preventing formation of all deoxyribonucleotides. Cells cannot make DNA and thus cannot divide. The dATP and adenosine accumulated leads to developmental arrest and apoptosis of lymphocytes.

2. When deoxyadenosine in lymphocytes accumulates leads if to inhibition of S-adenosylhomocysteine hydrolase, the important enzyme that has role in conventing S-Adenosylhomocysteine to homocysteine and adenosine. Excessive accumulation of S-adenosyl homocysteine in lymphocytes leads to premature apoptosis. Elevated adenosine levels lead to inappropriae activation of adenosine receptors. Adenosine is a signaling molecule and stimulation of the adenosine receptors results in protein kinase. Increased activity leading to increasing levels of cyclic AMP in thymocytes results in triggering of both apoptosis and developmental arrest of the cells.

Deficiency

1) **ADA**	2) **purine nucleoside phosphorylase**
Both T and	**T-cells affected,**
B-cells affected.	**B -cells are normal.**

- Immune dysfunction appear to result from accumulation of dGTP and dATP.
- These allosterically inhibits ribonucleotide- reductase, thereby decrease cells of DNA

Precursors, particularly dCTP.

HYPOURICEMIA.

Figure 4.3 Metabolism Changes in Gout

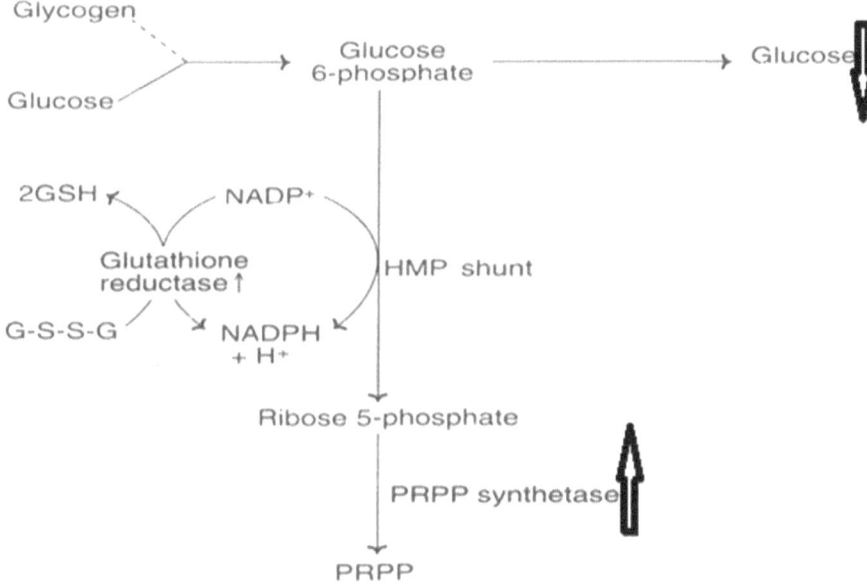

Palliative treatment:

- **Anti-inflammatory drugs:**
- **Colchicines'** is used. Others include **indomethacin, ibuprofen.**
- **Steroids** also used.
  gh

Pseudogout:

- Serum uric acid level *normal.*
- Symptoms as seen in gout.
- But it is characterized by deposition of **calcium –pyrophosphate crystals.**

Hypouricemia:

- Defective enzyme xanthine oxidase which is deficiency, either genetic or due to severe liver damage.
- Patients exhibit xanthinuria and xanthine lithiasis.

Chapter 5
PYRIMIDINES STRUCTURE AND METABOLISM

Transfer of ribose phosphate: This is transferred from PRPP, forming OMP (orotidylate), catalyzed **by orotate – phosphoribosyl transferase.**

Figure 5.1 pyrimidine structure

Thymin e2,4-dioxy 5methylpyrimidine

Cyto sin e 2-oxy 4 amino pyrimidine

Uracil 2,4 - dioxyp yrimid in e

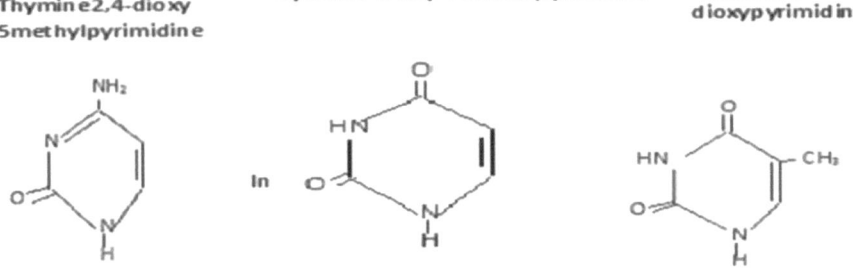

Denovo synthesis of pyrimidines
Orotic acid

orotate phsphoribosyl transferase OMP and OMP decarboxylase UMP PRPP is required in the conversion of orotic acid to orotidylic acid (OMP). OMP later on converted to CTP by series of reactions. Catalysed by different enzymes.
Features:

- Due to lack of feedback inhibition orotic acid. Production is excessive. (UMP inhibits OMP decarboxylase). Rapidly growing cells are affected resulting anemia. Retarded growth. Crystals excreted in urine cause blockage result in urinary obstruction. Both types respond to uridine, as it is converted to UTP. This acts as feedback inhibitor.

43

Other causes of orotic aciduria:

1. **Deficiency of liver mitochondrial ornthine – transcarbamoylase (X-linked).**

$$\downarrow$$

Under utilised substrate carbamoyl phosphate enters cytosol

$$\downarrow$$

Stimulates pyrimidine nucleotide biosynthesis

$$\downarrow$$

Leading to orotic aciduria

Disorders of pyrimidine metabolism:

1. **Orotic Aciduria:**

Orotic aciduria type I – deficiency of Orotatephosphoribosyl transferase and OMP –Decarboxylase.
Orotic aciduria type II:
Rare, deficeincy of only OMP decarboxylase.
Both types are inherited as **autosomal recessive** disorders.

2. **Drugs may precipitate orotic aciduria:**

a) **ALLOPURINOL,** a purine analog is a substrate for Orotate phosphoribosyl transferase.

$$\downarrow$$

It competes for phosphoribosylation with natural substrate, orotic aicd.

$$\downarrow$$

The resulting nucleotide product inhibits

$$\downarrow$$

OMP DECARBOXYLASE

$$\downarrow$$

Leading to Orotic aciduria

2. b) 6 – azauridine
It is Converted to 6-azauridylate

$$\downarrow$$

Competitively inhibits OMP decarboxylase

$$\downarrow$$

Enhancing excretion of orotic acid

3. Reye's syndrome:
Severely damaged liver mitochondria
↓
Carbamoyl phosphate is under utilised
↓
Enters into cytosol
↓
Leading to over production of orotic acid and
↓
Orotic aciduria.

Inhibitors of pyrimidine synthesis:

➢ **CTP** inhibits aspartate transcarbamoylase and prevents formation of carbamoyl aspartate (feed back inhibition) which is result of combing of Aspartate and Carbamyl phosphate.

➢ **5- Fluoro Uracil** inhibits the synthesis of thymidylate.

Chapter 6
REPLICATION

Replication

Watson and Crick noted that the structure of DNA itself suggested a mechanism for its replication. The copying process in which a single DNA molecule becomes two identical molecules is called **replication.** Simply it is doubling of DNA.

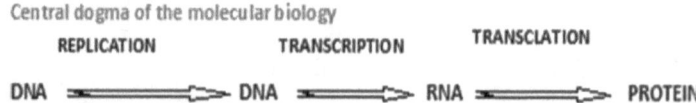

Central dogma of the molecular biology

REPLICATION   TRANSCRIPTION   TRANSCLATION

DNA ══════════▷ DNA ══════════▷ RNA ══════════▷ PROTEIN

<u>Histones</u>

- Parental Histones segregate conservatively during replication
- Old histones are enter leading daughter DNA duplex(ie they do not dissociate from the DNA during replication)
- Newly synthesized Histones become a part of the DNA containing the lagging strand
- Reason for this difference is Histones bind much more strongly to ds DNA than ss DNA

Introduction

Synthesis of daughter DNA by parent DNA during the cell division is called replication. In replication the genetic information is transmitted from the parent to offspring.

S phase; DNA replication takes place.

- *DNA replication occurs at polymerization rates of* about 500 nucleotides per second in bacteria and about 50 nucleotides per second in mammals.
- Clearly, the proteins that catalyze this process must be both accurate and fast.

- Speed and accuracy are achieved by means of a multienzyme complex that guides the process and constitutes an elaborate "replication machine.

Features:

- Replication occurs in **5' to 3'** direction only.
- Replication is **bidirectional.**
- Replication is **simultaneous** on both strands.
- Replication is **semi-conservative**.
- Replication **obeys base pair rule strands**
- Replication results in 2 daughter DNA strands.
- Each daughter DNA strand conserves half of parent strand and one complementary strand is synthesized newly. Hence this Replication is **semi-conservative**. Held by phospho-di-ester bonds and Hydrogen bonds

DNA synthesis begins at replication origins:

- Replication origin: The position at which the DNA is first opened.
- DNA polymerase *cannot start a completely new DNA strand*; it can join a new nucleotide only to a base-paired nucleotide in the double helix. Primer is very essential for initiation of replication.
- DNA polymerase can elongate a new DNA chain **only in the 5'-3' direction**.

Models for DNA REPLICATION:
These are many hypothesis to explain the process of replication. They are
1. Conservative model
2. Semi conservative model
3. Dispersive model

Requirements

1. Deoxyribonucleotides [dATP, dGTP, dCTP, dTTP]
2. Template DNA strand [parent strand]
3. RNA primer
4. Enzymes
   - **DNA polymerase**
   - **Primase**
   - **Helicase**

- **DNA Ligase**
- **Topo-isomerases**
- **Single Strand Binding Proteins.**

Single strand binding protein (SSBP)

O Binds to ssDNA
O Has two function
1. Prevents reannealing, thus exposing ss template required by polymerases is separate the two strands
2. Protects ssDNA from nuclease activity Show cooperative binding

Helicases

❖ Separate the ds DNA to ss DNA by dissolving the hydrogen bonds holding the two strands together
❖ These separates dsDNA at physiological temperature
❖ ATP dependent
❖ At least 9 helicases have been described to important role in E coli
❖ Of which DNA binding protein A, B, C (Dna A, Dna B, Dna C) are significant
❖ Is the Initial separator Dna A
❖ Continued further by Dna B (major strand separating protein acts bidirectionally)
❖ Dna C directs Dna B at site of replication

Helicase

Primase:

➤ Primase is a specialized RNA polymerase
➤ It synthesis a short strech of RNA in 5' to 3' direction on a template running in 3' to 5' direction.
➤ An RNA primer, about 100-200 nucleotides long, is synthesized by the RNA primase.
➤ The RNA primer, using exonuclease activity replaces with deoxyribo nucleotides by DNAP

DNA Ligases

DNA ligases ligates the DNA by close nicks in the phosphodiester backbone of DNA. Two of the most important biologically roles of DNA ligases are:

1. Joining of Okazaki fragments during replication.
2. Catalyzing short-patch DNA synthesis during in DNA repair process.

There are two classes of DNA ligases:
1. The first uses NAD^+ as a cofactor and only found in bacteria.
2. The second uses ATP as a cofactor and is present in eukaryotes, viruses and bacteriophages.

DNA Ligase Mechanism
The reaction occurs in three stages in all DNA ligases:

1. Formation of a covalent enzyme-AMP intermediate linked to a lysine side-chain in the enzyme and marks the first step in the mechanism.
2. Transfer of the AMP nucleotide to the 5'-phosphate of the nicked DNA strand.
3. Attack on the AMP-DNA bond by the 3'-OH of the nicked DNA sealing the phosphate backbone and resealing AMP.

Supercoils

➤ As two strands unwind, they result in the formation of positive supercoils (super twists) in the region of DNA ahead of replication fork.
➤ Accumulation of these supercoils interferes with further unwinding of ds DNA.
➤ This problem is solved by the enzyme **Topoisomerases.**
➤ These catalyze the interconversion of topoisomers of DNA

Catalyze in a three step process

1. Cleavage of one or both strands of DNA
2. Passage of a segment of DNA through this break
3. Resealing of the DNA

O Two types of topoisomerases are present
DNA which different in the linking numer
> Linking number = (Twist +Wreth) 3 dimentional

a. -type I topoisomerases
b. -type II topoisomerases

Topoisomerases I

✓ Reversibly cut one strand of double helix
✓ Have both nuclease (strand cutting) & ligase (strand resealing)
✓ Donot require ATP,rather use the energy released by phosphodiester bond cleavage to reseal the nick
✓ Removes only negative super coils
✓ Ex: bacteria

Topoisomerases II (DNA gyrase)

✓ Heterodimer with 2 swivelase & 2 ATPase subunits
✓ Swivelase subunit catalyzes trans esterification reaction that breaks & reforms the phosphodiester backbone
✓ ATPase subunit hydrolyzes ATP to trigger conformational changes that allow a double helix to pass through the transient gap
✓ Possitive super coiled

DNA polymerases

O These are the enzymes responsible for the polymerisation of deoxy ribo nucleosides, triphosphates on a DNA template strand to form a new complementary DNA strand.
O In prokaryotes based on site and conditions of action. They are divided into 3 types: I II III.

Common properties

1. All polymerases can synthesis a new strand of DNA in 5' to 3" direction. On a template strand which is running in 3'to 5' direction.
2. They also show Exo nuclease activity (it cleaves the end terminals of DNA) in 3'to 5' direction.
3. All DNA polymerases cannot initiate the process of replication on their own. This is the basic defect of DNAP synthesis of new strand.

Table 6.1 Comparison of prokaryotic & eukaryotic DNA polymerase and their functions

Prokaryotic	Eukaryotic	Function
	A	Gap filling & synthesis of lagging strand
II	E	DNA proofreading & repair
	B	DNA repair
	gamma	Mitochondrial DNA synthesis
III	Δ	Leading strand synthesis

Figure 6.1 Replication Fork

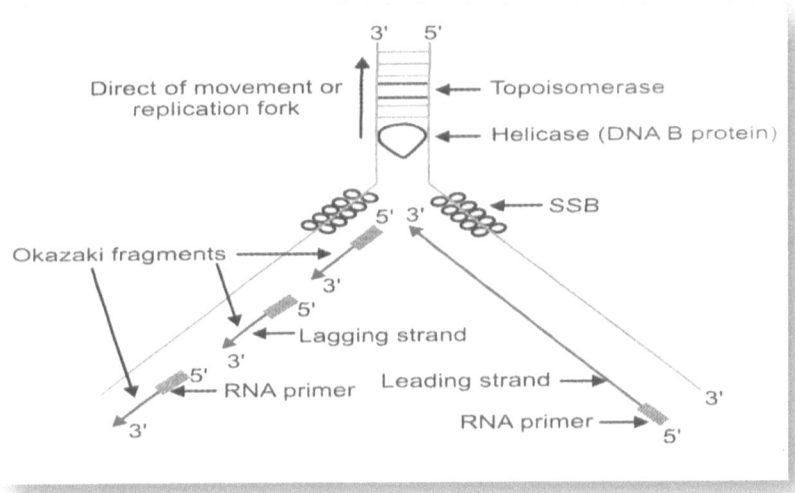

There are three phases of replication

1. Initiation
2. Elongation
3. Termination

Steps in DNA-replication:

1. **Initiation:**

Initiation site at which the replication is initiated is called initiation site. In bacteria the initiation site is called "Ori-C" site.

The ori-site consists of 245 basepairs. It is having some special features. They are It contains a tandom array of 3 thirteen meric sequence. or extreme left side these thirteen meric sequences are rich in A-T contents. The extreme right side is having four nonameric sequences. The DNA replication is initiated by a group of proteins **Dna A,B, C**

A specialized RNA polymerase called primase synthesis a short stretch of RNA in 5'- 3' direction on 3'-5' stand.

2. **Elonagation:**

In elongation the DNA polymerase III is positioned at the replication fork where it begins the synthesis of leading strand using RNA primer, formed by primase. The polymerase III does not leave the template untill replication has been completed. Synthesis on 3'-5' stand is continous.

The mode of synthesis of lagging strand is more complex. It is synthesized in fragments. So that direction 5'-3' polymerization leads to over all growth in 3'-5' directions. These fragments are called Okazaki fragments.

Okazaki fragments:

- ➢ The First demonstrated by Reiji Okazaki
- ➢ Short fragments of the DNA present on lagging strand resulted by the retrograde synthesis.
- ➢ The Okazaki fragments of human cells in average about 150 - 250 nucleotide in length

3. **Termination:**

Termination site is responsible for meeting both replication forks at exact opposite sites of Ori-C. Replication terminus is large region flanked by 6 nearly identical non palendromic sequence terminators sites.

The arrest of replication fork motion of ter sites sequences, the action of Tus proteins. These Tus proteins also binds with Dna B protein to inhibit its helicase activity. After termination the DNA'S are in catenated form. The 2 DNA's present in catenated structure are separated into 2 individual DNA'S by the action of DNA gyrase.

Replication inhibitors:

1. **Inhibitors of DNA**; To Prevents un-winding of DNA.
   E.g. Actinomycin and mitomycin

2. **2. Inhibitors of deoxy-ribonucleotides;**
   E.g. Anti-folates [inhibits Purine and Pyrimidine synthesis]

3. **3.Inhibitors of replicative enzymes**;
   E.g. Norflox [Inhibit the DNA gyrase]
   Ciploflox

Replication in Eukaryotic DNA (linear DNA)
The DNA molecules in Eukaryotic cell are considerably large than those in bacteria and are organized into complex nucleo protein structure (chromatic).
The essential feature of DNA replication are same in Eukaryotic and prokaryotics. However some interesting variations have been identified.

- ➤ The More complex than the prokaryotic replication
- ➤ The Semicoservative,occurs bidirectional from more oigins forming multiple of replication bubbles.
  - o Eg:- replication of the Drosophilia chromosomes
    - ▪ single Ori C ---16 days to replicate
  - o multiple Ori C ---3 min (6000 replication forks)
- ➤ The Sequence functionally similar to the Ori C have been identified in the yeast & are called as ARS (autonomously replicating sequence)
- ➤ Autonomously replicating sequence (ARS) –span about 300bp (conserved sequence)
- ➤ There are about 400 ARS elements in yeast

Table 6.3 The Eukaryotic of DNA polymerases

ROLL NO	Type DNA polymerases	Location	Major role
1	A	Nucleus	The Replication of nuclear DNA Gap filling & synthesis of lagging strand
2	B	Nucleus	Proof reading and Repair of nuclear DNA

3	Γ	**(Mitochondria)l**	Replication of mitochondrial in DNA
4	Δ	**Nucleus**	Replication of nuclear DNA Also Leading strand synthesis
5	E	**Nucleus**	Repair of the nuclear DNA

Polymerases:

✓ DNA-dependent DNA polymerases
    Eg. Prokaryotic and Eukaryotic DNA polymerases

✓ DNA-dependent RNA polymerases
    Eg. RNA polymerases and DNA primase

✓ RNA-dependent DNA polymerases
    Eg. Reverse transcriptase

✓ RNA-dependent RNA polymerases
    Eg. RNA replicase

Errors of Replication:

1. **Xeroderma Pigmentosum:** (It is an autosomal recessive genetic disorder. There is a defect of nucleotide excision repair in this condition).
   Important clinical features are: sensitivity of sunlight which causes blister on the skin. There is a risk of developing skin cancer and death occurs in the second decade of life.
2. **Hereditary Polyposis Colon cancer:** Caused by mutations in genes for proteins involved in mismatch repair (hMSH1,2 and hMSH3) (hPMS1 and hPMS2). The inability to repair mismatches increases the mutation frequency in growth regulatory genes.
3. **Melanoma:** 7 in 100,000 people (malignant melanoma) melanoma's develop from exposure of the skin to the Ultraviolet radiation (or) rays of the sun. The Ultraviolet radiation causes pyrimidine dimmers to forms in DNA. Resulting mutations may produce melanoma's appearing appear as dark brown growths on the skin.
4. **Nick "O" Tyne:** It has lung cancer, which accounts for one-fifth of cancer in men and 1/10 in women. The overall 5- year's survival rate is still < 15%. For those who smoke 2 or more packs of cigarettes daily, as does

Nick O Tyne, the risk of dying of lung cancer is > 22 times higher than for a non smokers.

5. **Also Ataxia Telngectasia and Cystic Fibrosis are errors of replication**

DNA REPAIR

The DNA repair majorly removed wrong base by DNA glycosylase and Endonuclease cuts the backbone near the defect (adjacent bases are removed). The gaps are filled by the correct bases by the action of DNA polymerase (repair enzyme) and DNA ligase.

DNA Damage (or) Mutation (or) changes in DNA

The main cause is base alteration by UV light irradiation and chain breaks by ionizing radiation and radioactive disintegration.

Mutation: Any change that occurs in DNA which is heritable is said to be "Mutation".

Mutaion are of 2 types 1.Chromosomal Mutation and 2. Gene Mutation.

Chromosomal Mutation: chromosomal have a definite structure and organization which is normally const from on mitosis to other. They however, sometimes under go certain structural modification which are known as chromosomal aberrations. Since these modifications also results in change of organism, they are also called chromosomal mutation. Chromosomal mutation should be distinguished from gene mutations. Gene mutations involve the changes only in single gene on the chromosome. Chromosomal mutation on the other hand usually results in changes in blocks of genes.

Chromosomal aberrations are 4 types

A) Deletion (or) Deficiency
B) Duplication
C) Inversion
D) Translocation

A. **Deletion (or) Deficiency:** Deletion involves loss of a chromosomal section. If a break takes place on a chromosome the part without centromere is lost, while the part with centromere functions as deficient chromosome. Deletions are 2 types 1. Terminal and 2 intestinal deletion.

1. **Terminal Deletion:** If a single break occurs near the end of chromosomes it results in terminal deletion.

2. **Intestinal Deletion:** In this case the breaks in the chromosome are followed by reunion of broken ends and the part between breaks is eliminated.

B.**Duplication:** In duplication a part of chromosome is present twice. ie; in duplicate. The nucleus therefore has extra chromosomal material beyond the normal chromosome compliment. Duplication are 2 types they are 1. Tandom duplication and 2. Reverse tandom duplication.

1. **Tandom Duplication:** Suppose a sequence of chromosomes in a chromosome is a b c d f g h I (Dot between e & f represent centromere) In tandom duplication the section of e is repeated immediately after its normal position.
2. **Reverse Tandom Duplication:** It involves a reversle of the duplicate segment i.e; a,b,c,d,e. e d f g h i

C. **Inversion:** In inversion the section of chromosome become changed by rotation through 180^0. The order of genes in the section is thus reversed. In this process only the arrangement of genes will change, not the no of genes.

D. **Translocation:** In translocation the segment of chromosome becomes attached to a non homogenous chromosomes. In translocation these is no addition or loss of genes, only rearrangement of gene takes place.

Gene Mutation: Classification

1. **Forword Mutation: A wild type of DNA on mutation gives different type of DNA.**
   A) **Mutation at DNA level**
      ➢ **Substitution (Transition and Transversion)**
      ➢ **Deletion**
      ➢ **Addition**
      ➢ **Inversion**
   B) **Mutation at protein level**
      ➢ **Silent mutation**
      ➢ **Missence mutation**
      ➢ **Frame shift mutation**

2. **Backward Mutation:**
   A mutant type of DNA converts into wild type of DNA
   - ➢ **Suppressor reversion mutation**
   - ➢ **Exact reversion mutation**
   - ➢ **Equivalent reversion mutation**

Mutations of DNA level:

Substitution: In this type of mutation incorporation of a wrong base takes place during replication or repair. substitutions are of 2 types they are 1. Transition and 2. Transverion

Transition: If one purine base is replaced by another purine base {A/G or G/A} or a pyramidine base {T/C or C/T} are known as transition.

Transverion: If a purine base is replaced by a pyramidine base or viceversa it is called "Transversion". Total for four bases of DNA we have four transitions and 8 transversions.

Mutations leading to base pair substitution presumely in 2 types.

Let us consider a mutation in a DNA duplex strand in which the purine "A" base is replaced by "G" after on replication if it give rise to 2 DNA duplexes one normal like parent DNA and the other is mutant.

Inversion: If a segment of DNA is removed & reinsert in reverse direction it results in inversion. So, the message is in out of phase only in the triplet involved is the inversion.

Fame shift mutation: A mutation in which there is deletion or insertion of one a few nucleotides it is called a frame shift mutation. The name is derived from the fact that there is a shift in the reading frame either in backward or forward direction by one or two nucleotides. It is obtained by the following bases.

Deletion: Removal of one or two bases from a nucleotide chain is called deletion. If will be seen that the removal of even are base will throw the genetic message out of frame beyond the point of deletion.

Insertion: Adding of one or few additional bases to the nucleotide chain leads to shifting of genetic message. If there is simultaneous deletion and addition of bases then the message will be out if frame only in the triplet between deletion and addition.

Silent Mutation: Any gene mutation which does not result change in phenotypic expression is called silent mutation. The genetic code is degenerative i.e. more than on codon may specify an amino acid for example; Both AAG and AAA specify

Lysine. If the Codon AAG undergoes a mutation to AAA the latter codon still specify lysine. When the mutated triplet codes for the same amino acid as the original there is no change in amino acid. This mutation is of final type because although these is a change in base sequence of DNA, there is no alteration in the amino acid sequence of protein synthesized. The codon changed may result in an amino acid substitution but this is not sufficient to modify the function of protein appreciably. The mutation may occur in gene i.e; no longer functional a whose protein is not essential at the particular stage of testing.

Missense Mutation: A missense mutation is one which results in the replacement of one amino acid in a polypeptide chain by another. As a result of mutation one base of codon [May then code for another amino acid] may be substituted by another base the changed codon may the code for another amino acid. A missense mutation can be caused by substitution deletion or insertion. Missense mutation arising by a substitution results in proteins which differ from a normal counter parts only in sing amino acids. Such proteins therefore frequently have normal biological activity. Example: On of the codon for phenylalanine is GUU; A single base substitution U to G changes it to UGU codes for cystein. Thus the protein formed after mutation is identical to the normal protein except the phenyl alanine is substituted by cysteine.

Suppressor Mutation: The effect of a mutation in the phenotype can be reversed so that the original wild type phenotype is brought back. This reversal may be due to reversion (or) suppression. In a true reversion there is a reversal of the original genetic information. A C to A mutation would change the codon GCU (alanine) to GAU Aspartic acid. This may result in the enzyme form becoming inactive. In a true reversion a reverse mutation from A to C would restore the codon for Alanine (GAU to GCU). Mutation due to suppression are 2 types they are 1. Intragenic suppression and 2. Intergenica suppression

1. **Intragenic suppression:** the codon that has undergone a change as a result of mutation may undergo another mutation to a codon that is less harmful to enzyme function. Thus mutation of GCU (Alanine) to GAU (Aspartic acid) may result in an inactive enzyme. A second mutation A to U would give the codon GUU for valine and they may restore the enzymatic activity partially or fully.

2. **Intergenic suppression:** If the deleterious effect of a mutation in a gene is overcome by a mutation in another gene then it is called intergenic suppression.

Leaky Mutation: If a mutation has taken place from "X" to "Y" that "Y" is not going to affect the function of total protein. But it can reduce the effect of protein.

Table 6.4 Techniques in Molecular Biology

SNO:	TECHNIQUE	SAMPLE ANALYSED	PURPOSE
1	Karyoptyping	Chromosomes	chromosomal anamalies
2	DNA Sequencing	DNA	Knowledge of Genetic Code & Mutations.
3	RFLP & SOUTHERN BLOTTING	DNA	Polymorphism, Mutations.
4	NORTHERN BLOTTING	mRNA	Amount & size of mRNA.
5	WESTERN BLOTTING	Proteins	Protein of Interest can be isolated.
6	FISH	DNA	Diagnosis of Disease & Prognosis
7	PCR	DNA	Detection at early stage of Disease
8	DNA Microarrays	DNA	Detects changes in GENE Expression.
9	DNA Finger Printing	DNA	Potent Weapon in Forensic Medicine.
10	Recombinant DNA	DNA	Production of Therapeutic Proteins
11	GENE Library	DNA	Search for a specific GENE is made easy

Chapter 7
TRANSCRIPTION

Formation of RNA by nuclear DNA is called as transcription. In gene expression, transcription is the beginning step. In this, a portion of the double-stranded DNA template gives rise to a single-stranded RNA molecule. In some cases, the RNA molecule itself is a "finished product" that serves the important functions within the cell. Often, however, transcription of an RNA molecule is followed by translation step, which ultimately results in production of a protein molecule. DNA is double-stranded between the two strands only one strand serves as a template for transcription at any given time. This template strand is called the noncoding strand. The non template strand is referred to as the coding strand because its sequence will be the same as that of the new RNA molecule. Almost in all organisms, the strand of DNA that serves as the template for one gene may be the non-template strand for other genes within the same chromosome. During transcription, a DNA sequence is read by an enzyme known as RNA polymerase, which produces a complementary, antiparallel RNA strand called a primary transcript.

Similarities between replication and transcription are in terms of chemical mechanism, polarity, and use of template but difference is, it does not require primers and requires only a short segment of DNA that is transcribed.

All 3 types of cellular RNA's are transcribed during transcription.
- Messenger RNAs (mRNAs) encode the amino acid sequence of one or more polypeptides specified by a gene or set of genes.
- Transfer RNAs (tRNAs) read the information encoded in the mRNA and transfer the appropriate amino acid to a growing polypeptide chain during protein synthesis.
- Ribosomal RNAs (rRNAs) are constituents of ribosomes, the intricate cellular machines that synthesize proteins.

Transcription- Requirements

- SsDNA-act as template
- DNA dependent RNA polymerase
- Regulatory proteins
- Ribonucleoside triphosphates (ATP, GTP,CTP, UTP)
- Sigma factor
- Rho factor

Steps involved in Transcription
Initiation:

The first step in the initiation of transcription is recognition and binding of RNA polymerase to the promoter site.

The RNA polymerase finds promoters by searches process, in which low affinity (loose complex) and then moves along the DNA until it reaches a promoter sequence to which it binds with higher affinity (tight complex) the sigma factor is required for the formation of this thight complex. After the recognition of -35 sequence by RNA polymerase the unwinding of DNA takes place at -10 base sequence (open Complex).

Once the DNA open the RNA polymerase starts synthesising at zero. When 2 bases are added at zero amd 1 then that complex is called "Terenary complex"

Until 9 bases are added the RNA polymerase will not move as well as sigma factor doesn't leave the core enzyme. Elongation is performed only by core enzyme after sigma factor has left it.

Strand Elongation

When transcription is initiated, the DNA double helix unwinds the strand and RNA polymerase reads the template strand, adding nucleotides to the 3' end of the growing chain.

RNA Polymerase(E.Coli)

Dr.Grander discovered RNA polymerase. The RNA polymerase do not have Exonuclease activity. RNA polymerase is present in cytoplasm and it is Multisubunit enzyme.

DNA dependent RNA polymerase is Very large molecule (500 kd) and complex enzyme consisting of four kinds of subunits and molecular weight 490,00. RNA polymerase helps synthesis of (mRNA, t RNA, r RNA) and it detects the terminating signals also interacts with the transcription factors.

- They are 5 types ($\alpha_2\beta\beta'\ \Omega\sigma$ ------holoenzyme)

RNA polymerase with out σ subunit is called core enzyme and Core enzyme contains the catalytic activity. The core enzyme can transcribe a DNA duplex after transcription has been initiates at proper site. The core enzyme has 4 polypeptides like $\alpha_2\beta\beta'\Omega$ polypeptides. Sigma factor is loosely held with RNA poly it recognizes certain specific sequence and DNA template and binds RNA poly unit.

Table 7.1 RNA polymerase gene and function

Subunit	Gene	Number	Mass (kd)	Role
A	rpo A	2	37	Binds regulatory proteins
β	rpo B	1	151	Forms phosphodieter bond
β'	rpo C	1	155	Binds DNA template
σ	rpo D	1	70	Recognizes promoter & initiates synthesis

Termination

Because of the great stability of transcription complex, termination of transcription with the release of nascent transcript is a an complex process.

In bacteria there are 2 types of termination mechanisms

They arreree

1. Rho factor independent termination mechanism
2. Rho factor dependent termination mechanism

Rho factor moves towards 3' end, displacing the between temperature and transcript making them to dissociate. Combined action of Rho factor and secondary structure removes RNA polymerase. Later Rho factor also be removed giving free primary RNA transcript.

Genes with strong promoters cause frequent initiation of transcription as often as every two seconds (E coli – strong promoters have sequence that correspond closely to the consensus sequence).Genes with weak promoters are transcribed about once in 10 minute (weak promotes tend to have multiple substitution at that site).

Inhibitors of Transcription (Mostly antibiotics)

1. Actinomycin-D (DNA strand blocks)
2. Rifampicin (Anti tuberculosis)
3. Alpha Amanitin (Inactivate RNA polymerase II)

4. Mitomycin (Intercalate with DNA strands and prevent the transcription)
5. Streptomycin (This specifically inhibits chain elongation by the prokaryotic type of RNA polymerase).

The hnRNA is called heterogeneous nuclear RNA. It is a precursor form of mRNA, formed as native RNA in the nucleus as primary transcript. It's molecular weight is $>10^7$ where as Mol.Wt. of mRNA is $<2 \times 10^6$. On further processing it is converted to mRNA.

Post-transcriptional Modification

In the post-transcriptional modification the processing of RNA primary transcript occurs primarily within nucleus. It's aim is mainly to protect from exonucleases activity. It is not needed in prokaryote because its half life is very short.
Important points in post-transcriptional modification are:

- ✓ Nucleolytic and ligation reactions splicing of exons ()
- ✓ Terminal additions (addition of cap and Poly 'A' tail in mRNA and attachment of CCA terminal to the tRNA).
- ✓ Nucleoside modification: Methylation; deamination to produce unusual bases.

The hnRNA undergoes post-transcriptional modification to form mRNA. The following changes take place during post-transcriptional modification.

- ➤ Addition of cap by a 7 methyl GTP at 5 hydroxytermius.
- ➤ Attachment of poly 'A' tail consisting of 20-250 nucleotides in length at 3 hydroxy terminus.
- ➤ Internal nucleotides are methylated. Methylation takes place at N_6 of adenine residues and 2 hydroxy group of ribose.
- ➤ Splicing: The hnRNA has two types of sequences of nucleotides.

    1) Exons: These are the sequence of coding region of DNA. These are transcribed into proteins.
    2) Introns: These are the non coding region of DNA. These are nontranscribed into a protiens

Removal of noncoding sequence by joining adjacent exons is called splicing. Splicing carried out by cutting out of introns sequence and joining the ends of neigh boring exons to produce a functional mRNA. Afterwords the mRNA molecule is transported to cytoplasm. A berent splicing causes some forms of Thalasemia.

Chapter 8
TRANSLATION

The synthesis of protein molecule is a cell by arranging the amino acids in a sequence bond is called protein synthesis.

Requirements for protein synthesis:

1. mRNA
2. tRNA
3. Ribosomes
4. Aminoacids
5. Translational factor
6. Energy (ATP and GTP)
7. eiF (Eukaryotic Initiation Factors)
8. TheVarious inorganic cations like (e.g. K^+, NH^+ and Mg^{2+}).
9. Blue print for the construction of – DNA nucleotide sequence. (Genetic code)

The mechanism of protein synthesis can be divided into the following 3 main steps in prokaryotes and eukaryotes.

1. Initiation
2. Elongation
3. Termination

The main steps of initiation are:

A) Binding of mRNA to ribosomes.
B) Selection of initiation codon.
C) Activator of amino acid.

The steps elongation includes:

A) Joining two aminoacids by peptide bond formation.
B) Moving the mRNA and ribosomes with respect to one another.

The steps of termination include:

A) Dissociation of polypeptide chain that is completed, from the synthetic mechinary.
B) Release of ribosomes to begin another side of protein synthesis.

Ribosomes: The mRNA and tRNA interact together on the ribosomes and translate the message into a specific protein molecule. Ribosome in E.Coli is large 70S complex of both protein and rRNA, consisting of 50S and 30S subunit.

1. 50 S subunit contains 23S RNA, 5S RNA and 34 proteins
2. 30S subunit contains 16 S RNA and 21 proteins.

Topography: The Topography of ribosomes shows that it contains an mRNA of the ribosomes site and 3' 16S rRNA and 30S subunits.

P-Site by binds with the A site
S-Site peptidyl of the tRNA binds.

Initiation:
Shine Dalgarno sequence is present 10-13 bases upstream to initiation codon. This sequence is recognized by a small subunit of ribosome with its 16S RNA. The association of larger subunit to smaller subunit is prevented by the IF-III that binds to smaller subunit of ribosome. So IF-III is named as "anti- association factor". Smaller subunit occupied shine dulgarno sequence along with AUG as "P" site occupies initiation codon. Now the IF-II brings aminoacyl tRNA (having an initiate code that is methionated) especially to "P" site by using GTP. The tRNA which is coding for another AUG other than initiator AUG is different. IF-III will be dissociated. Now the larger subunit will come & attached to smaller subunit. IF – I stabilize the subunits of ribosome.

Elongation:
The elongation refers addition of the aminoacids one by one to first aminoacid is methionine, as per refers to the sequence codon in the mRNA. Codon of mRNA is the recognises and for the recognition aminoacyl-tRNA containing the corresponding anticodon moves to words 70S ribosome and fits into A-site. Here the anticodon of tRNA base pair with a second codon of mRNA.

The peptide bond is formed between carboxyl group (COOH) of the first amino acid of site-P and amino group (NH_2) of the second amino acid is A-site. Peptide bond links two amino acids to the frame a dipeptide. Bonding is catalyzed by enzyme peptidyl transferase present in the 50S ribosomal subunit. After the formation is peptide bond, methionine and the tRNA are separated by the enzyme called as a tRNA deacylase.

Dissociated of the 1st tRNA is released from P-site into cytoplasm for the further amnioacylation. Now the ribosomes moves on mRNA into 5' to 3' direction so that first codon goes out of the ribosomes, second codon comes to the lie in P site from A site and third codon comes to lie into A site. Simultaneously, second tRNA is the shifted from A site to the P site. All these events, movement of second tRNA from A site to P site constitute translocation. The translocation is catalysed by enzyme is called translocase. The third codon is the recognized and aminoacyl tRNA containing for the corresponding anticodon moves to 70S ribosome and fits into A site. Anticodon base pair with the codon.

Peptide bond is the formed between third amino acid is site A and second amino acid of the dipeptide present in Psite. Thus a tripeptide is formed. Then ribosome moves into 5' to 3' direction. Second tRNA and second amino acids are dissociated. The second tRNA is released from the P site into cytoplasm.

Amino acids are added on by the one as per therefore codon in mRNA and hence this tripeptide converted into the polypeptide chain. Polypeptide chains elongate by addition of more and more amino acids.

Elongation of the polypeptide chain is brought about by the a number of protein factors called as elongation factors. Three elongation factors in the prokaryotes, they are called as elongation factor **EF-Ts, EF Tu and EF-G**. In eukaryotes, they are called EfI beta, EFI gama and EF-2. Ribosomes reaches about 25th codon on to the mRNA. A new ribosome gets attached into the initiation codon and starts from synthesizing another polypeptide chain. In this way of many ribosomes are moving on a mRNA. Cluster of the ribosomes on an mRNA is called as a polyribosome. Each ribosome carries a growing of polypeptide chain. Each ribosome synthesizes a polypeptide chain, each mRNA is also used to synthesizes more copies of polypeptide chains.

Termination:

1.   tRNA's for stop codons –UAA,UGA and UAG not exist
     •   protein releasing factor recognizes stop codons.
     •   RF I is recognizes UAA and UAG

- RFII is recognizes UAA and UGA
- 16 S rRNA is essential in reading the stop codon.

2. Binding of RF to the terminating codons causes water to accept the growing peptide.
3. Release of peptide is followed by
   - Dissociation of mRNA and tRNA
   - Dissociation of 30S and 50S subunits
   - Binding of IF3 to 30S subunit to prevent reassembles in the absence of mRNA and fmet-tRNA.

Eukaryotic translation:

Eukaryotes don't have Shine dulgarno sequence is not present in eukaryotes. Smaller subunits of ribosome finds 5'cap of mRNA & seans the codons whatever the AUG it reaches first while seaning is initiation factor. Here initiation factor are indicated as eIFS. eiF -4 facilitates binding of smaller subunit to cap. eiF-I,II,and eiF III,have same function as in prokaryotes. But around 14 eiF are there.

Inhibitors of protein synthesis: Reversible inhibitors (bactreiostatic)

1. Puromycin (antibiotic) in block A site
2. Strepto mycin (block the inhibition canbe formation & block protein synthesis)
3. Chloramphinical (it inhibit peptydyl transvesion)
4. Tetracycline: (binds to 30S subunit ribosome& inhibit binds of aminoacyl RNA to A site)

In Eukaryotes:

1. Puromycin (structural analog of tyrosinyl tRNA and causes premature termination of proteins.)
2. Cyclocheximide
3. Diptheria toxin(The fragment 'A' of diphtheria toxin causes transfer of ADP-ribose moiety from NAD to EF2 and inhibits protein synthesis).
4. Ricin (Inactivates 28s rRNA and prevents protein synthesis).

Post translational modification:

The native protein further undergoes modification after termination. The native protein in the form of preproprotein is converted to actual protein by the removal of pre and pro peptides and it may further undergoes hydroxylation, Glycosylation, Methylation, carboxylation, and acetylation reactions to form actual protein.

The native proteins in the form of pre-pro insulin and pre-pro collagen are converted to insulin and collagen by the following mechanism;

- In the pre-pro insulin the pre sequence of amino acids are called leader sequence consisting of 23 amino acids and pro sequence has 35 amino acids and actual insulin has 51 aminoacids.
- Modification of amino acid gamma carboxylation of glutamic acid residues of prothrombin.
- Glycosylation –addition of glucose.
- Hydroxylation- lycine in collagen
- Phosphorylation- addition phosphate (PK), Removal phosphate (P.Phosphate)

Genetic code: The relationship between sequence of bases in DNA or RNA and the sequence of amino acid in a polypeptide chain is called genetic code. The code indicates that which codon specify which amino acid. A recapitulation of the relationship between genes and proteins is desirable for understanding the genetic code.

- All metabolic reaction are catalyzed by specific enzyme (proteins)

- The action of an enzyme depends upon the sequence of amino acids constituting it

- The one gene- one enzyme hypothesis proposed by Beedle & Talum in 1940 states the synthesis of an enzyme (actually of a polypeptide chain is controlled by a particular gene).

- The gene which is almost always a segment of DNA strand, transcribes an mRNA strand, which intern translates a polypeptide chain.

- Messenger RNA thus acts as an intermediate in conveying information from the sequence of nucleotides in DNA to the sequence of amino acids in the polypeptide chain (sequence hypothesis)

- Each amino acid is specified by a sequence of there bases (the codon on mRNA)

- Each tRNA molecule has a sequence of three bases (the anticodon) which reads a codon of m RNA, tRNA molecule these serves as adoptor in protein synthesis by reading mRNA codons in a sequence (cricks adaptor hypothesis)

1. **Amino acids involved in protein synthesis:**
   About 150 aminoacids found in nature of which only 20 aminoacids are specified by the genetic code. Only these 20 aminoacids take part in protein synthesis. Among the other aminoacids found in proteins are cystine (a double aminoacids consisting of two cysteine molecules) and hydroxy proline (formed by addition of hydroxyl group to proline). A polypeptide chain typically consists of 100-300 aminoacids & is formed by specific arrangement of 20 types of amino acids.

2. **Genetic code is triplet code:** DNA contains four (ATG&C) protein are synthesized from 20 different types of amino acids. A basic problem ariase regarding genetic code was how many bases of DNA specify on aminoacid. In a singlet code, each DNA or letter would specify one amino acid. In two letter codon is concerned it specify only (4x4) 16 amino acids. A triplet code was first suggested by physicist **GAMOW** according to him (4x4x4= 64) it specifies 64 amino acids. The triplets are called codons. Since these are 64 codon & only 20 amino acids each aminoacid may be called by more than one codon i.e. the code is degenerative.

3. **Genetic code and overlapping:** Since the DNA molecule is along chain of nucleotide it could be read either in a overlapping or nonoverlapping manner. The genetic code thus be overlapping or non overlapping. The reading of code by these two different ways yield two different results. In non overlapping code six nucleotides would code of two amino acids while in the overlapping code it can be read three times each time as a part of different word. Mutation changes in on e letter would effect only on word in non overlapping while it would effect three words in the overlapping code.

4. **Genetic code is Commaless:** All the available evidence indicate that the code is commaless, that is there are no demarcinating signals between them. The work of **KHORONA** cited below gives a clear evidence of a commaless code. Long synthetic polypeptide nucleotide with specific repeating sequence were used for translation of a protein chains. These the separating sequence CUCUCU..contains the codon CUC (for Leucine) & UCU(for serine). When this sequence is used for translation of proteins, either amino acid is incorporated into the protein unless the other is also present. This results can only be explained by a commaless triplet code where these would have to be atending tranloaction of CUC & UCU codons).

5. **Degeneracy of codon:** There are 64 possible codons in a triplet code of which 61 have been shown to code aminoacids since only 20 amino acids takes place in protein synthesis it is obvious that these are many codons than amino acid type. So it is obvious that more than one codon codes for same amino acid. Degeneracy of codons associated with tRNA. If you consider 5' AUG 3' codon that pairs an anticodon 3' UAC 5' (anti codon should be read from reverse side i.e. 5' to 3'). Degeneracy of codon is best explained by Wobble hypothesis by Crick.

6. **Wobble Hypothesis:** Wobble means loose it was proposed by Crick. According to wobble hypothesis, only the first two positions of a triplet codon on a mRNA have a precise pairing with the bases of the tRNA anticodon.

   • The pairing of 3rd positions of bases of the codon maybe ambigious is & varies according to the nucleotide present in this position.

   • Such interaction between the 3rd bases referred to as wobble pairing (totally the pairing between 3rd base of codon & 1st base of anticodon is not obligate i.e. mismatching is seen). The pairing of first base of anticodon is not obligate if A pairs with U, if U pairs with A or G.

   • Inosine to U,C& A i.e. Thus a single tRNA type is able to recognize two or more codons differing only in the 3rd base example: the anticodon UCG of serine tRNA recognizes two codons AGC & AGU.

   • The bonding between UCG & AGC follows the usual Watson & Crick pairing pattern. In UCG –AGC pairing however hydrogen bonding takes place between G & U.

   • This is a departure from the usual Watson & Crick pairing (pattern) mechanism where G pairs with C & A with U mRNA codon (serine).

   • The degeneracy of the code is not random mostly the different codon for a particular amino acid base the same first letters (Leucine, Serine, & Arginine are exceptions). Thus the first two letters of all the four codons for valine are GU & for Alanine GC.

7. **Genetic code is nearly universal (Non Ambigious):** The genetic code is valid for all organisms ranging from bacteria to man it is essentially the same for all organisms and is therefore said to be universal. The universality of the

code was demonstrated by Marshall, cascade and Hirenberg, who found that E.Coli (bacterium) Xenopus laevis (amphibians) and Guinea pig (mammals). Amino acyl t RNA use almost all the same code this shows that essentially universal.

Chapter 9
GENE THERAPY

Gene therapy is an experiment technique that uses genes to treat or prevent disease. It is the intracellular delivery of genes to generate a therapeutic effect by correcting an existing abnormally. Gene therapy offers a chance of a correcting such fatal disease.

Gene therapy offers is the process of inserting genes into cells to treat disease. The newly introduced genes will encode proteins and correct the deficiencies that occur in genetic disease. Thus, genes therapy primary involves genetic manipulation in animals or humans to correct a disease, and keep the organism in good health.

In the future, this technique may allow the doctor to treat a disorder by inserting a gene into a patient's cells instead of using drug or surgery.

Researchers are testing several approaches to gene therapy, including;

Replacing a mutated gene that causes disease with a healthy copy of the gene. Inactivating or knocking out a matured gene that is functioning improperly. Introducing a new gene into the body to help fight a disease. Although gene therapy is a promising treatment option for a number of diseases (including inherited disorders, some type of cancer and certain viral infections).

The technique remains risky and is still under study to make sure that it will be safe and effective. Gene therapy is currently only being tested for the treatment of disease that have no other cures.

Every person's gene are different, and the changes in sequence determine the inherited difference between each of us some changes usually in a single gene, may cause serious disease (such as cystic fibrosis, muscular dystrophy, and thalassemia). More often, gene variant interacts with the environment to predispose some people to cancer or heart disease or other common ailments.

Gene augmentation therapy, a DNA is inserted into the genome to replace the missing gene product. In the case of gene inhibition therapy, the antisense gene inhibits the expression of the dominant cells.

Our cells are divided into 2 groups, the (somatic cells which make up working parts of the body, and the germ cells (or sex cells; sperm in men and eggs in women) which pass on genetic material to our children.

Every normal somatic cell contains the same coded DNA. Instruction, even if only some of them are used. Different ones will be active different parts of the body. If a body cell is modified by

Two types they are somatic and germ cell:

1. Somatic cell

In somatic cell gene therapy (SCGT), the therapeutic genes are transferred into any of any cell other than a gamete, germ cell, gametocyte or undifferentiated stem cell. Any such modifications affect the individual patient only and are not inherited by offspring. Somatic gene therapy represents mainstream basic and clinical research, in which therapeutic DNA (either integrated into the genome or as an external episome or plasmid) is used to treat disease.

Gene disorders are good candidates for somatic cell therapy. The complete correction of a genetic disorder or the replacement of multiple genes is not yet possible. Only a few of the trials are in the advanced stages.

2. Germline

In germline gene therapy (GGT), germ cells (sperm or eggs) are modified by the introduction of functional genes into their genomes. Modifying a germ cell causes all the organism's cells to contain the modified gene. The change is, therefore, heritable and passed on to later generations. Australia, Canada, Germany, Israel, Switzerland and the Netherlands prohibit GGT for application in human beings, for technical and ethical reasons, including insufficient knowledge about possible risks to future generations and higher risks versus SCGT The US has no federal controls specifically addressing human genetic modification (beyond FDA regulations for therapies in general

Vector

Vectors in gene therapy

The delivery of DNA into cells can be accomplished by multiple methods. The two major classes are recombinant viruses (sometimes called biological nanoparticles or viral vectors) and naked DNA or DNA complexes (non-viral methods).

Viruses (viral vector)

In order to replicate, viruses introduce their genetic material into the host cell, tricking the host's cellular machinery into using it as blueprints for viral proteins. Scientists exploit this by substituting a virus's genetic material with therapeutic DNA. (The term 'DNA' may be an oversimplification, as some viruses contain RNA, and gene therapy could take this form as well.) A number of viruses have been used for human gene therapy, including retrovirus, adenovirus, lentivirus, herpes simplex, vaccinia and Adeno-associated virus. Like the genetic material (DNA or RNA) in viruses, therapeutic DNA can be designed to simply serve as a temporary blueprint that is degraded naturally or (at least theoretically) to enter the host's genome, becoming a permanent part of the host's DNA in infected cells.

Non-viral

Non-viral methods present certain advantages over viral methods, such as large scale production and low host immunogenicity. However, non-viral methods initially produced lower levels of transfection and gene expression and thus lower therapeutic efficacy. Later technology remedied this deficiency.

Methods for non-viral gene therapy include the injection of naked DNA, electrophoresis the gene gun, sonoporation, magnetoreception, the use of oligonucleotides, lipoplexes, dendrimers, and inorganic nanoparticles.

Hurdles

- Short lived nature is on of the unsolved problems- Before gene therapy can become a permanent cure for the a condition, therapeutic DNA introduced into the target cells must be functional and cells containing to therapeutic DNA must for stable.
- Immune response – The Anytime a foreign object is introduced into the human tissues, immune system is stimulated to the attack for invader. Stimulating of immune system in a way that the reduces gene therapy effectiveness is possible. The immune system's enhanced response to the viruses that it has seen before the reducing effectiveness to the repeated treatments. The problems with the viral vectors- Viral vectors carry

risks of toxicity, inflammatory responses, gene control and targeting issues.

- The Multigene disorders like commonly occurring disorders, such as the heart disease, high blood pressure, Alzheimer's disease, arthritis, and diabetes, are affected by the variations in multiple genes, which complicate gene therapy.

- Insertional mutagenesis – If DNA is the integrated into a sensitive spot in genome, for the example in a tumor suppressor gene, Therapy could induce a tumor. This has occurred in the clinical trials of X-linked severe combined immunodeficiency (X-SCID) patients, in which hematopoietic stem cells were transduced with the corrective transgene using a retrovirus, and this is led to development T cell leukemia in the 3 of 20 patients. The one possible solution is to add a functional tumor suppressor gene to DNA to be integrated. This may be problematic since longer DNA is the harder it is to the integrate into cell genomes. CRISPR technology allows for researchers to make much more precise genome changes at the exact locations.

Functional Classification:

- Base on the purpose of gene therapy it can be
- Gene replacement therapy
- Gene deactivation therapy
- Transgenesis
- Gene Enhancement therapy
- Gene activation therapy

Somatic cells or the Germ line cells are the cells to accept the introduced genes.
- ➤ Based on the type of cells involved the Gene therapy can be-
- ➤ Somatic cell therapy
- ➤ Germ line therapy

1) **Germline Gene Therapy**
   Normal version of gene is inserted into germ cells
   a. those germ cells will divide normal versions of the gene
   b. any zygote produced as a result of this germ cell will have a correct version of the defective gene and will continue passing it on to *their* offspring.
2) **Somatic Cell Gene Therapy**
   Single defective cell is taken out of an individual's body

Functional version of gene introduced into cell in a laboratory

a. cells reproduce
b. copies of cells with a corrected version of the gene is injected back into the patient

The good gene ends with the patient and is not inherited by their offspring

Introduce the genes:

There are three ways-

➢ *Ex vivo* strategy- Where the patients cells are cultured in the laboratory, the new genes are infused into the cells and modified genes are administered back to the patient

➢ *In situ strategy*- where the carrier of the gene is injected to the patient either intravenously or directly to the tissues.

➢ *In vivo* strategy- where the vector is administered directly to the cell.

Isolate the healthy gene along with its regulatory sequence to control its expression. Incorporate this gene on to a vector or carrier as an expression cassette. Deliver the vector to the target cells.

Vectors role in gene therapy:

➢ Different carrier systems are used for gene delivery-
➢ 1) Viral systems
➢ 2) Non-viral systems
➢ Vectors are needed since the genetic material has to be transferred across the cell membrane and preferably into the cell nucleus.

Viral vectors:

1) Retroviruses
2) Adenoviruses
3) Adeno associated viruses
4) Herpes simplex viruses

NON-VIRAL SYSTEMS:

1) Spontaneous uptake by endocytosis
2) Plasmid liposome complex
3) Uncovered plasmids
4) Gene gun methods

5) Electroporation
6) Microinjections.

Non-viral approach- liposome
Retroviruses:

The retroviruses are modified to carry genes. The *gag, pol, Env* genes are deleted rendering them incapable of replication inside the host cell. Viruses are then introduced into a culture containing the helper viruses. The helper virus is an engineered virus which is deficient in Ψ segment but contains all other genes for replication. That means it has the genes to produce viral particles but lacks the genes required for packing.

Retroviruses as vectors:

The replication deficient but infective retrovirus vector carrying the human gene now comes out of the cultured cells. These are introduced into the patient. The virus enters the cell via specific receptors. In the cytoplasm of the human cells, the reverse transcriptase carried by the vector converts the RNA into DNA, Which is then integrated into the host DNA. The normal human gene can now be expressed. The integrated DNA becomes a permanent part of the chromosome.

Advantages and Disadvantages:

> As he virus is deficient in replication, so it's safe and is suitable as per the treatment of a variety of diseases. Cancer gene therapy involves into introduction of tumor cell containing the genes for cytokine into patients. Introduction of tumor suppressor gene into the patients is an alternative method for cancer gene therapy. Some gene therapy protocols are used in the genetic immunization or DNA vaccines.
> May be disrupted by normal genes
> Rapidly dividing cells are used as targets by retroviruses the non-dividing cells cannot be used.

Adeno associated virus and Herpes simplex virus:

- **Adeno associated virus:** It is also a DNA virus. Which has no known pathogenic effect and has wide of tissue affinity. It integrates at the a specific site.
- **Herpes simplex virus:** This is a disabled single copy of virus that is defective glycoprotein. When propagated into complementary cells, viral

particles are generated. Since they can be replicate only once so there is for no risk of the disease.

Accomplishments of Gene Therapy:

- **Severe combined Immunodeficiency (SCID):** It is caused by deficiency of the adenosine Deaminase enzyme. It was the first trial of gene therapy done on this disease. The follow-up studies shows presence of the normal immune functions for recipients compatible with the life.

- ✓ Restenosis – 13 patients were treated by the DNA carrying genes for angiogenesis. All were improved.
- ✓ Breast cancer, prostate cancer, lung cancer, brain cancers and ovarian cancers have been treated.
- ✓ The activation of Hb F gene in the patients of Thalassemia and sickle cell diseases.
- ✓ Trials for enhance into the genes of intelligence, height, and athleticism.
- ✓ Trials to treat individuals with the genetic predisposition to conditions such as the asthma, alcoholism and Alzheimer's disease. Schizophrenia, manic depression and Breast cancer before the onset for clinical manifestations.

Targets for gene therapy:

o **Genetic disorders:**
1) Duchenne Muscular dystrophy
2) Cystic fibrosis
3) Familial hypercholesterolemia
4) Hemophilia
5) Haemoglobinopathies
6) Gaucher's disease
7) Albinism
8) Phenylketonuria.

Acquired diseases:

- Cancers
- Infectious disease- HIV

- Neurological disorders
- Cardiovascular diseases
- Rheumatoid arthritis
- Diabetes mellitus

Ethical Issues:

- Who decides what is normal and what is a defect
- What kind of an impact will this have on people who are currently living with these disabilities? Will this make them feel worse about themselves?
- Gene therapy is expensive so will only the rich have access to treatment? What will happen to the poor?
- It is possible that gene therapy given to an adult could reverse a genetic disease. If so, would that therapy also prevent any children the person had after gene therapy from inheriting the disease?

Figure 9.1 Gene therapy and disease

Serial No:	DISEASE	GENE THERAPY
1	Severe combined immunodeficiency (SCID)	Adenine Deaminase (ADA)
2	Cystic fibrosis	Cystic fibrosis trans membrane regulator(CFTR)
3	Familial hypercholesterolemia	Low-density lipoprotein (LDL) receptor
4	Emphysema	Alfa 1 antitrypsin
5	Hemophilia B	Factor IX
6	Thalassemia	Alfa or Beta globulin
7	Sickle- cell anemia	Beta globulin
8	Lesch-Nyhan syndrome	HGPRT
9	Gaucher's disease	Glucocerebrosidase
10	Peripheral artery disease	Vascular endothelial growth factor(VEGF)
11	Fan conin anemia	Fan conin anemia
12	Melanoma	Tumor necrosis Factor (TNF)
13	Melanoma renal cancer	Interleukin -2 (IL-2)

14	Glioblastoma (brain tumor) AIDS ovarian cancer	Thymidine kinase (herpes simplex virus)
15	Head and neck cancer	P53
16	Brest cancer	Multidrug resistance 1
17	AIDS	Rev and env
18	Colorectal cancer, melanoma, renal cancer	Histocompatibility locus Ag –B7 (HLA-B7)
19	Duchenne muscular dystrophy	Dystrophy
20	Short stature	Growth hormone
21	Diabetes	Glucose transporter -2 (GLUT-2) glucokinase
22	Phenylketonuria	Phenylalanine hydroxylase
23	Citrullinemia	Arginosuccinate synthetase

Chapter 10
PHYSICAL MAPPING OF GENOMES

The Gene mapping, also called **genome mapping**, this creation of the genetic map of assigning DNA fragments to the chromosomes.

When a genome is the first investigated, it is a map nonexistent. Map improves with scientific progress and is the perfect when a genomic DNA sequencing of species has been completed. During this process, and this investigation of differences in the strain, Fragments were identified by small tags. These may be genetic markers (PCR products) or Unique sequence-dependent pattern for DNA-cutting enzymes. Ordering is the derived their genetic observations (recombinant frequency) for these markers or Second case from the computational integration for fingerprinting data. The term "mapping" is used also two different but related contexts.

The two different ways of mapping are distinguished. Genetic mapping uses classical genetic techniques (e.g. pedigree analysis or breeding experiments) determine sequence for features within the a genome. Using for modern molecular biology techniques of same purpose is the usually referred to the physical mapping.

Mapping the Genome:

Human genome project hasbeen provided us with the draft of a ***entire human genome***.

- 4 Bases: A, T, C, G
- 3.12 billion of base-pairs
- 99% of these are same
- *Polymorphisms* = where they differ

Physical Mapping

The physical mapping, DNA is cut by the **restriction enzyme**.

Possible to reconstruct for order of the fragments from the sizes of the fragments{3,5,5,9}

Gel Electrophoresis: Example

This resulting pattern for DNA migration (i.e., its genetic fingerprint) is used to the identify what stretch of DNA is clone. By analyzing of fingerprints, contigs are assembled by the automated (FPC) or manual means (Pathfinders) into the overlapping DNA stretches. The macrorestriction is the type for physical mapping wherein high molecular weight DNA is digested with the restriction enzyme having a low number of restriction sites.

The alternative ways to determine how DNA in a group of clones overlaps without completely sequencing for clones. Once the map was determined, Clones can be used as a resource to the efficiently contain large stretches for genome. This type is mapping of more accurate than genetic maps.

The genes can be mapped prior to complete the sequencing by the independent approaches like of in situ hybridization. Genetic maps serve to guide a scientist toward a gene, just like an interstate map guides a driver from city to city. Physical maps are more similar to street maps and allow a scientist to more easily home in on a gene's location.

This scenario is similar to situation facing scientists searching for the specific gene for somewhere within vast human genome. They have available to them two broad categories of maps: **genetic maps** and **physical maps**

PHYSICAL MAPS

Types of Physical Maps and What They Measure

Physical maps can be divided into three general types: **chromosomal** or **cytogenetic maps**, **radiation hybrid (RH) maps**, and **sequence maps**. The different types of maps vary in their degree of **resolution**, that is, the ability to measure the separation of elements that are close together. The higher the resolution, the better the picture.

The lowest-resolution physical map is the chromosomal or **cytogenetic map**, which is based on the distinctive banding patterns observed by light microscopy of stained chromosomes. As with genetic linkage mapping, the chromosomal mapping can be used to locate genetic markers defined by traits observable only in whole organisms. Because chromosomal maps are based on estimates of physical distance, they are considered to be physical maps. Yet, the number of base pairs within a band can only be estimated.

RH maps and sequence maps, on the other hand, are more detailed. RH maps are similar to linkage maps in that they show estimates of the distance between genetic and physical markers, but that is where the similarity ends. **RH maps** are able to provide more precise information regarding the distance between markers than can a linkage map.

The physical map that provides the most detail is the sequence map. **Sequence maps** show genetic markers, as well as the sequence between the markers, measured in base pairs.

How Are Physical Maps Made and Used?

RH Mapping

RH mapping, like linkage mapping, shows an estimated distance between genetic markers. But, rather than relying on natural recombination to separate two markers, scientists use breaks induced by radiation to determine the distance between two markers. In RH mapping, a scientist exposes DNA to measured doses of radiation, and in doing so, controls the average distance between breaks in a chromosome. By varying the degree of radiation exposure to the DNA, a scientist can induce breaks between two markers that are very close together. The ability to separate closely linked markers allows scientists to produce more detailed maps. RH mapping provides a way to localize almost any genetic marker, as well as other genomic fragments, to a defined map position, and RH maps are extremely useful for ordering markers in regions where highly **polymorphic genetic markers** are scarce.

Scientists also use RH maps as a bridge between linkage maps and sequence maps. In doing so, they have been able to more easily identify the location(s) of genes involved in diseases such as spinal muscular atrophy.

Chapter 11
GENETIC EXPRESSION

Introduction:

- *Genetic expression* is a process by the which inheritable information from a gene, such as DNA sequence, is the made into a functional gene product, such as the protein or RNA
- The non-protein-coding genes (e.g. rRNA genes, tRNA genes) are transcribed, they are not translated into protein.
- Controlled expression for genetic information requires the multitude of factors that interact specifically and non-specifically with the DNA.
- Expression of the Genetic information in a given cell or organism, Synthesis of RNA and proteins specified by the DNA sequence is note either random fully preprogrammed
- Process of regulation for gene expression generally involves a interaction of specific binding proteins with the various regions of DNA in the immediate vicinity of transcription start site (positive or negative effect).
    1. Enhancement or silencing.
    2. Tissue-specific expression.
    3. Regulation by Hormones, metals and chemicals

The addition to transcription level control, gene expression also modulated by

- ➢ Gene amplification
- ➢ Gene rearrangement
- ➢ Post-transcriptional modification and
- ➢ RNA stabilization
- ➢ Genome organization

Regulation of Gene expression is required for Development, Differentiation and Adaptation:

- The two types for Gene regulation (Positive and Negative regulation)
- When the expression of genetic information is the quantitatively increased in the presence of a specific for regularity element then the regulation is said to be **positive**.
- When the expression of genetic information is diminished by presence of the specific regulatory element, regulation is the said to be **negative**.
- Element or molecule mediation negative regulation is said to be the negative regulator or repressor, that is mediating positive regulation for positive **regulator** or **activator**.

Gene expression in Prokaryotes:

- The group of organisms that lack to cell nucleus or any other membrane-bound organelles.
- The differ from eukaryotes, which have the cell nucleus
- Mode of division is the binary fission
- The prokaryotes exhibit efficient genetic mechanisms to be respond to environmental conditions

Types of genes in Gene Expression

- Inducible gene: The Regulated by inducer/activator
- Constitutive gene: Not subjected to the regulation

Regulation of Prokaryotic Gene Expression:

- The control at the level of **transcription**
- The high rate of the mRNA turnover in prokaryotes also serves to change the metabolic machinery very quickly in response to the various microenvironments.
- *Induction* - Production of a specific enzymes in response to the presence of a substrate
- *Repression* - Cessation of production of a specific enzymes in response to an increased level of a substrate.
- All of the genes which the encode for enzymes necessary for this pathway are found next to each other on the *E. coli* chromosome

- The single mRNA carries of information for the multiple proteins
- This type of the mRNA is called a ***polycistronic mRNA*** and is totally unique to the prokaryotes

Operon Models

- The operon model is also self-regulating series for genes found on to DNA that work in concert
- This includes the special segment of genes that regulators of the protein synthesis but *do not code* for protein, called the **promoter** and **operator** regions
- Lactose (Lac), Tryptophan (Trp) and L-Arabinose (Ara)

Lac Operon Model

- ❖ The Inducible system
- ❖ 3 genes part of the operon that code for the three separate enzymes
- ❖ Those needed for the breakdown of lactose, a simple sugar

The E-Coli lac OPERON:

- OPERON - Genes of lactose metabolism.
    - z - gene codes for β-galactosidase
    - y - gene for lactose permease
    - x - gene for trans acetylase

Table 11. 1: Lac Operon gene functions

	Lac Operon Gene	Gene Function
1	**Lac I**	Constitutive gene synthesizing repressor constantly
2	**Lac Z**	Gene for β-galactosidase subunit
3	**Lac Y**	Gene for Permease subunit
4	**Lac A**	Gene for Thiogalactoside transacetylase subunit
5	**Promoter or P**	RNA polymerase binding & initiator of transcription
6	**Operator or O**	Repressor binding site

In addition regularity, the gene coding for lac repressor is located in a separate locus for the lac operon.

Components of Lac Operon:

- Lac operon repressed when E.Coli grows in Glucose and Lactose containing a medium.
- Lac genes are derepressed or activated only after the glucose has been depleted for the medium.
- The expression of the lac operon was controlled by both a negative repression system and a positive activator system.

Lac I		Promoter gene	Operator gene	Lac Z	Lac Y	Lac A

Repression System

- Lac Operon negatively controlled by repressor a protein that binds to DNA operator site and inhibits transcription.
- In the presence of inducer, the repressor binds to induce and change the confirmation of repressor so that it cannot binds to operate the site.

Activator System

- ➤ In addition to the inducer, lac operon also regulated by a positive control element whose presence is essential for transcription.
- ➤ Positive control elements – cAMP – CAP complex
    (Catabolite gene – activating protein)
- ➤ When Glucose presence in the media, the levels of cAMP are low.
- ➤ When Glucose utilized completely in the media, the cAMP levels elevated.
- ➤ cAMP binds to CAP – CAP binding site.
- ➤ cAMP – CAP complex facilitates the binding of RNA polymerase to the lac promoter results in transcription of the lac operon genes.
- ➤ Repression of the lac-OPERON genes by the presence of **glucose – Catabolite repression**.

Trp Operon Model
The top operon

An example is a *trp* gene in **bacteria**. When there is a high level of **tryptophan** in the region, the bacterium may not want to synthesize more because it wants to save energy. When the **RNA polymerase** binds and transcribes the *trp* gene, the **ribosome** will start translating. (This differs from eukaryotic cells, where RNA must exit the nucleus before translation starts.) The attenuator sequence, which is located between the mRNA leader sequence (**5' UTR**) and trp operon gene sequence, contains four domains, where domain 3 can pair with domain 2 or domain 4.

The attenuator sequence at domain 1 contains instruction for **peptide** synthesis that requires tryptophans. A high level of tryptophan will permit ribosomes to translate the attenuator sequence domains 1 and 2, allowing domains 3 and 4 to form a hairpin structure, which results in termination of transcription of the trp operon. Since the protein-coding genes are not transcribed due to rho-independent termination, no tryptophan is synthesized.

P/O	Trp L		TrpE	Trp D	Trp C	Trp B	Trp A

In contrast, the low level for tryptophan means that is ribosome will stall at domain 1, and causes the domains 2 and 3 to form the different hairpin structure that does not a signal termination of transcription. Therefore rest for a operon will be transcribed and translated and tryptophan can be produced. Thus, domain 4 is an attenuator. Without domain 4, translation can be continue regardless of level of the tryptophan. Attenuator sequence has its codons translated into the leader peptide but is not part of trp operon gene sequence. Attenuator allows more time for this attenuator sequence domains to the form loop structures but does not produce of protein that is also used in later tryptophan synthesis.

Attenuation is the second mechanism for negative feedback of trp operon. The TrpR **repressor** decreases transcription by the factor of 70 and attenuation can be further decrease it by the factor for 10, ther by allowing accumulated repression of about 700-fold. The attenuation is made up possible by fact that in prokaryotes (which have no nucleus), ribosomes begin translating a mRNA while RNA polymerase is the still transcribing DNA sequence. This allows a process of translation to the directly affect to transcription of operon.

Table 11.2: Tryptophan operon gene functions

Trp Operon Gene	Gene function
P/O	Promoter; operator sequence is found in the promoter
Trp L	Leader sequence; attenuator (A) sequence is found in the leader

Trp E	Gene for anthranilate synthetase subunit
Trp D	Gene for anthranilate synthetase subunit
Trp C	Gene for glycerol-phosphate synthetase
Trp B	Gene for tryptophan synthetase subunit
Trp A	Gene for tryptophan synthetase subunit

At beginning their transcribed genes of trp operon was the sequence of 140 nucleotides termed a leader transcript (trpL). There is transcript includes for four short sequences designated 1-4. Sequence 1 is the partially complementary to sequence 2, which is the partially complementary to sequence 3, which is the partially complementary to sequence 4. Thus, three distinct secondary structures (hairpins) can be form 1-2, 2-3 or 3-4. Hybridization for strands 1 and 2 to form 1-2 structure that prevents the formation of 2-3 structure while the formation of 2-3 prevents the formation of 3-4. The 3-4 structure of transcription termination sequence as and when it is forms RNA polymerase will be disassociate from DNA and transcription of the structural genes of the operon will not occur.

Part of leader transcript codes for the short polypeptide of 14 amino acids termed to the leader peptide. Peptide contains two the adjacent tryptophan residues, which is the unusual since tryptophan is the fairly uncommon amino acid (about one in the hundred residues in a typical E. coli protein is a tryptophan). Ribosome attempts to the translate this peptide while tryptophan levels of cell are low, it will stall at either of two trp codons. While it is stalled, ribosome physically shields sequence 1 of transcript, Preventing it forming the 1-2 secondary structure. Sequence 2 is then the free to hybridize with sequence 3 to form a 2-3 structure, which then prevents to the formation of 3-4 termination hairpin. RNA polymerase is alos free to the continue transcribing a entire operon. If the tryptophan levels of cell are high, this ribosome will translate the entire leader peptide without any interruption and will only stall during translation termination at this stop codon. At that point, Ribosome physically shields both the sequences 1, 2. Sequences 3 and 4 are thus free to form the 3-4 structure which terminates transcription. The end result is that operon will be transcribed only when the tryptophan was unavailable for the ribosome, while the trpL transcript is constitutively expressed.

In order to ensure that the ribosome binds and begins translation of the leader transcript immediately following its synthesis there is a pause which site exists in the trpL sequence. Upon reaching this site, RNA polymerase pauses transcription and apparently waits for the translation to begin. This mechanism allows of synchronization for the transcription and translation, a key element in the attenuation.

A similar attenuation mechanism regulates for synthesis of **the histidine, phenylalanine**, and **threonine.**

Proposed mechanism of the how this mRNA secondary structure and trp leader peptide could be regulate transcription for trp biosynthetic enzymes includes of the following.

- The RNAP initiates transcription for trp promoter.
- The RNAP pauses at about nucleotide 90 at the secondary structure (first one shown above).
- Ribosomes engage this is nascent mRNA and the initiate translation of the leader peptide.
- The RNAP is then "released" from the its pause and continues transcription.
- When RNAP reaches a region of the potential terminator, whether it could continues or not is dependent on to position of the ribosome "trailing behind".

Other operons controlled by attenuation

Dische overy of this type of the mechanism to a control of the expression of genes in the biosynthetic operon lead to the rediscovery in a wide variety of such as operons for twhich repressors had to never been discovered.

For example:

Operon	Leader peptide
Histidine	MTRVQFKHHHHHHHHPD stop
Threonine	MKRISTTITTTITITTGNGAG stop
Ilv (GEDA)	MTALLRVISLVVISVVVIIIPPCGAALGRGKA stop
IlvB	MTTSMLNAKLLPTAPSAAVVVVRVVVVVGNAP stop
Leucine	MSHIVRFTGLLLLNAFIVRGRPVGGIQH stop
Phenylalanine	MKHIPFFFAFFFTFP stop

Attenuation in Eukaryotes

Research conducted on microRNA processing showed an evidence of attenuation process in **Eucaryotes**. After co-transcriptional endonucleolytic cleavage by Drosha 5'->3' exonuclease XRN2 may terminate further transcription by torpedo mechanism.

Attenuation control of the histidine operon.

Histidine operon leader is an RNA element found in the bacterial histidine operon. At least 6 amino acid operons are known to be a regulated by the attenuation. In each, the leader sequence of 150-200 bp is found upstream of first gene in operon. This leader sequence can be assume two different secondary structures known as the terminator and anti-terminator structure. In each case, a leader also can codes of very short peptide sequence that is rich in end product amino acid of the operon. Terminator structure is the recognized as the termination signal of RNA polymerase and operon is not transcribed. The structure forms when this cell has been an excess of the regulatory amino acid and ribosome movement over the leader transcript is not impeded. When there is the deficiency of charged tRNA of the regulatory amino acid a ribosome translating to the leader peptide stalls and antitermination structure can form. This allows RNA polymerase to transcribe the operon.

Regulation of L-arabinose operon in the *Escherichia coli*

The genetic analysis of series for genetic experiments of increasing rigour and elegance, Englesberg, and his collaborators then the provided rather convincing evidence that the primary activity of AraC protein was in inducing a expression of the other arabinose specific proteins, AraC acted positively to turn on expression rather than acting negatively to turn off expression like *lac* repressor turns off the expression of the *lac* operon. That means that the intrinsic set state of *ara*-specific promoters is off and AraC turns them on, whereas the set state of *lac* operon promoter is on and *lac* repressor turns it off. Subsequently, definitive biochemical experiments proved that indeed, AraC acted positively to turn on expression for promoter that is serves to the *araB*, *araA* and *araD* genes

REGULATION OF GENE EXPRESSION IN EUKARYOTES

Special features are involved in regulation of eukaryotic gene expression
Most of the DNA in prokaryotic cells is organized into genes.
A very different situation exists in mammalian cells, in which relatively little of the total DNA is organized into genes

> ➢ Genome organisation
> ➢ Enhancers/ repressors
> ➢ Gene amplification
> ➢ Gene rearrangements
> ➢ RNA processing
> ➢ Regulation of mRNA stabilization

Chapter 12
DNA EXTRACTION
AND ISOLATION

Introduction

In this activity, you will extract a mass of DNA from bacterial cells visible to the naked eye.

1. The preparation of DNA from any cell type, bacterial or human, involves the same general steps:
    (a) Disrupting the cell (and nuclear membrane, if applicable),
    (b) Removing proteins that entwine the DNA and other cell debris, and
    (c) Doing a final purification.
        (i) These steps can be accomplished in several different ways, but are much simpler than expected. The method chosen generally depends upon how pure the final DNA sample is and how accessible the DNA is within the cell.
        (ii) Bacterial DNA is protected only by the cell wall and cell membrane; there is no nuclear membrane as in eukaryotic cells. Therefore, the membrane can be disrupted by using dishwashing detergent, which dissolves the phospholipid membrane, just as detergent dissolves fats from a frying pan. (The process of breaking open a cell is called cell lysis.) As the cell membranes dissolve, the cell contents flow out, forming a soup of nucleic acid, dissolved membranes, cell proteins, and other cell contents, which is referred to as a cell lysate. Additional treatment is required for cells with walls, such as plant cells and bacterial cells that have thicker, more protective cell walls (such as Gram-positive or acid-fast organisms). Additional treatments may include enzymatic digestion of the cell wall or physical disruption by means such as blending, sonication, or grinding.

2. After cell lysis, the next step involves purifying the DNA by removing proteins (histones) from the nucleic acid. Treatment with protein-digesting enzymes (proteinases) and/or extractions with the organic solvent phenol are 2 common methods of protein removal. Because proteins dissolve in the solvent but DNA does not, and because the solvent and water do not mix, the DNA can be physically separated from the solvent and proteins.
3. In this activity, you will not attempt any DNA purification: your goal is simply to see the DNA. You will lyse *E. coli* with detergent and layer a small amount of alcohol on top of the cell lysate. Because DNA is insoluble in alcohol, it will form a white, web-like mass (precipitate) where the alcohol and water layers meet. Moving a glass rod up and down through the layers allows you to collect the precipitated DNA. But this DNA is very impure, mixed with cell debris and protein fibers.
4. Before you begin the DNA isolation, make sure you know the procedure to follow. Draw out a flow chart below including the amount of each reagent and the time for that part of the procedure.

Materials

Disposable test tubes	Stock cultures	Water bath set at 60–70°C
Deionized water Dishwashing detergent (50% mixture) Glass rod	*E. coli*	Ice bath

Methods:

1. Apply your PPE, including eye protection, for this lab. Locate the water baths and the ice-cold ethanol.
    Determine a method for timing the various steps.
2. Label a 5-mL disposable tube and fill it with exactly 3 mL of distilled water. Using a swab, inoculate *E. coli* from the stock culture and agitate it in the 3 mL of distilled water.
3. Add 3 mL of the detergent to the suspension of *E.coli*. Mix each tube by gently shaking.
4. Place each tube into the water bath for 15 minutes. Maintain the water bath temperature above 60°C but below 70°C. A temperature higher than 60°C is needed to destroy the enzymes that degrade DNA.
5. Cool the tube in an ice bath until it reaches room temperature.

6. The next step involves precipitating the DNA by using solvent. Carefully pipete 3 mL of ice-cold ethanol (it may be in the freezer) on top of the detergent and *E. coli* suspension mixture. The alcohol should float on top and not mix. (It will mix if you stir it or squirt it in too fast, so be careful.) Water-soluble DNA is insoluble in alcohol and precipitates when it comes in contact with it.
7. By carefully placing a clean glass rod through the alcohol into the suspension, a web-like mass will become evident; this mass is precipitated DNA.

NOTE

The rod carries a little alcohol into the suspension, precipitating and attaching to the DNA. Do not totally mix the 2 layers.

DNA Isolation

DNA is isolated by a rapid non enzymatic method by salting out the cellular proteins by dehydration and precipitation with saturated sodium chloride solution.
Aim: Isolation of Genomic DNA from venous blood collected in EDTA
Equipment

1. Centrifuge
2. Microcentrifuge
3. Spectrophotometer
4. Electrophoresis Unit
5. DC power supply and Speed Vac or incubator

Procedure

1. 2 ml of blood is drawn in EDTA vaccutainers, mix well by inverting the tube and stored at 4°C till use.
2. Bring the blood sample to room temperature. Then transfer 2 ml of blood into a 15ml centrifuge tube and add equal volume of TKMI buffer.
3. Add 40 µl of Triton – X to lyse the red cells. Mix well by inversion
4. Centrifuge at 3000 rpm for 10 minutes at room temperature (RT) in a Beckman table top centrifuge.
5. Slowly pour off the supernatant and save the nuclear pellet (the small pellet settled at the bottom of the tube) and wash the pellet in 2 ml of TKMI buffer and centrifuge as before. Repeat the step if lysis is incomplete.

6. Add 320μl of TKM2 to the pellet and re-suspend the cells.
7. Add 50 μl of 10% SDS to lyse the WBCs and mix the whole suspension thoroughly and incubate for 10 min at 55°D. Later transfer the contents to sterile eppendroff tube.
8. Add 120 μl of 6M NaCI to the tube and mix well to precipitate the proteins by inversion and centrifuge at 12000 rpm for 5 min in a microcentrifuge.
9. Save the supernatant containing DNA and discard the pellet containing precipitated protein.
10. Transfer the supernatant to an eppendorf tube and add 2 volumes of 100% ethanol at room temperature. Invert the tube several times slowly till the DNA precipitates.
11. Centrifuge at 12000 rpm and discard the supernatant and add 1 ml of ice cold 70% ethanol.
12. Microcentrifuge the sample for 5 min at 12000 rpm at 4°C.
13. Dry the pellet in speed vacc or in an incubator. Resuspend DNA in 500 μl of Tris EDTA buffer at 65° C for 15 mins.

Preparation of Reagents (Approx for 50 blood samples)
TKMI buffer (500 ml)
Tris Hcl (10mM)pH 7.7 - 0.605g
KCI (10mM) - 0.372g
MgC12 (10mM) - 1.016g
EDTA (2mM) - 0.372g

TKM2 buffer (100ml) pH 7.6
Tris Hcl (10mM)pH 7.7 - 0.121g
KCI (10mM) - 0.073g
MgC12 (10mM) - 1.102g
EDTA (2mM) - 0.467g
NaC1 (0.4M0 - 0.467g
SDS (10%) – 1 gm of sodium dodecyl sulphate in 10 ml of doubled distilled autoclaved water
6 M NaC1 - 8.765 gms of NaC1 in 25 ml of distilled water
T.E. buffer (25ml) Tris HCl - (10mM)pH 3.0 - 0.030g
EDTA (1mM) - 0.009g
For the preparation of TKMI and TKM2 buffers the pH should be maintained by dissolving Tris in a few ml of water. The pH is maintained 7.6 by adjusting it

with 1% HC1. After maintaining the pH, EDTA is dissolved first and then the rest of the chemicals. The same procedure is followed also for TE buffer.

Estimation of DNA

The isolated DNA needs to be studied for its quality and quantity before using it in molecular biology experiments. Estimation is of two types

1. Quantitative
2. Qualitative estimation

Nucleic acid (DNA and RNA) has maximum absorbance at 260 nm. One OD value (Standard) corresponds approximately 50 µg/ml of double stranded DNA, 40 µg/ml of single stranded DNA/RNA and 20 µg/ml of oligonucleotides.

The ratio between the readings at 260 nm and 280 nm (OD 260/OD 280) provides an estimate of the purity of nucleic acid. Pure preparations of DNA and RNA have a ratio of approximately 1.8 and 2.0 respectively. If the DNA is contaminated with protein the ratio will be < 1.8 and the ratio is > 2.0 indicates that the DNA is contaminated with RNA. 5

Requirements:

DNA sample(s)

TE buffer (10mM Tris HC1 (pH 7.5): 1mM EDTA (pH 8.0)) / Sterile water

Spectrophotometer and Cuvetts

Quantitative Estimation
Protocol:

1. Add 10 µl of each isolated DNA sample to 2490 µl of TE buffer / sterile distilled water, (this corresponds to 250 fold dilutions), mix well and measure the absorbance at 260nm and 280 nm in the spectrophotometer to determine the quality and quantity of DNA
2. Calculate the concentration of DNA in the sample by the following formula: Amount of DNA (µg/ml) = Dilution factor x standard (50µl/ml) x OD at 260 nm
3. Calculate the ratio of absorbance between 260nm and 280 nm
   a. If the ratio is 1.8 to 2.0 the sample of DNA is relatively pure
   b. If the ratio is < 1.8 the sample of DNA is either contaminated with Phenol or Protein
   c. If the ratio is > 2.0 the sample of DNA is contaminated with RNA

Chapter 13
DNA FINGER PRINTING

The chemical structure of everyone's DNA is the same. The only difference between people (or any animal) is the order of the **base pairs**. There are so many millions of base pairs in each person's DNA that every person has a different sequence.

Using these sequences, every person could be identified solely by the sequence of their base pairs. However, because there are so many millions of base pairs, the task would be very time-consuming. Instead, scientists are able to use a shorter method, because of repeating patterns in DNA.

These patterns do not, however, give an individual "fingerprint," but they are able to determine whether two DNA samples are from the same person, related people, or non-related people. Scientists use a small number of sequences of DNA that are known to vary among individuals a great deal, and analyze those to get a certain probability of a match.

DNA Fingerprinting procedure:
Southern Blot

The Southern Blot is one of the way to analyze the genetic patterns which thee appear in a person's DNA. Performing thee Southern Blot involves:
The original mehod of blotting was developed by Suthern for detecting fragments in the agarose gel that ar complementary to a given DNA sequence.

Procedure: The DNA iis cut into fragments by using restriction enzymes and loaded on ta an agarose gel and allowted to restriction and agarose gel is mounted on a filter paper wick which dips into a reservoir containing "Transfer buffer".

The hybridization membrane (Nitro cellulose membrane) is sandwiched between the gel and a stock of paper towels (or other absorbant material) which serves to draw the transfer buffer through the gel by capillary action.

The DNA molecule are carried out of the gel by the buffer flow and immobilized on the membrane. (The membrane doesn't allow DNA to diffuse out but allows buffer). Generally used membrane material is Nitrocellulose. The main draw back with this membrane is its fragile nature and more over it fires at high temparture (80^0C).

For efficient southern blotting, gel pretreatment is larger DNA fragments (>10Kb require a long transfer time than short fragments to allow uniform transfer of a wide range of DNA fragment sizes, the electrophoresis DNA is exposed to a short depurination treatment by using alkali. This shortens the DNA fragments by alkaline hydrolysis at depurinated sites. It also denatureres the fragments prior to transfer ensuring that they are in single stranded state and accessible for probing. Finally the gel is equilibrated in neutralizing solution prior to blotting.

An alternative method uses positively charged nylon membranes. (as DNA is negatively charged) instead of normal membranes.

Alter transfer the nucleic acids are fixed to the membranes by baking the membrane is a vaccum oven at 80^0C.

Following the fixation step, the membrane is placed in a solution of labeled. (Radio active or non radio active but mositly radioactive) RNA or single strandad DNA, or oligo Deoxy nucleotides which is complementary in sequence to the blot transferred DNA band.

After the hybridization, the membrane is washed to remove unbound radioactivity and regions of hybridization are dectected by autoradiography

Making a Radioactive Probe

1. Obtain some **DNA polymerase** [pink]. Put the DNA to be made radioactive (radiolabeled) into a tube.
2. Introduce nicks, or horizontal breaks along a strand, into the DNA you want to radiolabel. At the same time, add individual nucleotides to the nicked DNA, one of which, *C [light blue], is radioactive.
3. Add the DNA polymerase [pink] to the tube with the nicked DNA and the individual nucleotides. The DNA polymerase will become immediately attracted to the nicks in the DNA and attempt to repair the DNA, starting from the 5' end and moving toward the 3' end.

4. The DNA polymerase [pink] begins repairing the nicked DNA. It destroys all the existing bonds in front of it and places the new nucleotides, gathered from the individual nucleotides mixed in the tube, behind it. Whenever a G base is read in the lower strand, a radioactive *C [light blue] base is placed in the new strand. In this fashion, the nicked strand, as it is repaired by the DNA polymerase, is made radioactive by the inclusion of radioactive *C bases.

5. The nicked DNA is then heated, splitting the two strands of DNA apart. This creates single-stranded radioactive and non-radioactive pieces. The radioactive DNA, now called a probe [light blue], is ready for use.

Practical Applications of DNA Fingerprinting

- 1. **Paternity and Maternity**
  Because the person inherits his or her VNTRs from his or her parents, VNTR patterns can used to the establish paternity and maternity. Patterns of so specific that the parental VNTR pattern can reconstructed even if only the children's VNTR patterns of known (more children produced, more reliable the reconstruction). Parent-child VNTR pattern analysis has been used to the solve standard father-identification cases as well as mony complicated cases for confirming legal nationality and, in instances of the adoption, biological parenthood.

- 2. **Criminal Identification and Forensics**
  The DNA isolated from blood, hair, skin cells, or other genetic evidence left at that scene of the crime can compared, through VNTR patterns, with DNA for criminal suspect to the determine guilt or innocence. VNTR patterns are also useful in the establishing the identity of the homicide victim, either from the DNA found as a evidence or from body itself.

- 3. **Personal Identification**
  Notion of using DNA fingerprints as a sort of genetic bar code to the identify individuals has been discussed, but this is not likely to happen for anytime in the foreseeable future. The technology required to the isolate, keep on file, and then analyze millions of very specified VNTR patterns is both the expensive and impractical. Social security numbers, picture ID, and other more mundane methods are much more likely to remain the prevalent ways to the establish personal identification.

Chapter 14
CLONING

Cloning is the creation of genetically identical cells (or) organisms from a single ancestral cell. Gene cloning refers to production of multiple copies of desired gene. Gene cloning procedure: Production of multiple copies of desired gene involves the following steps;

1. Isolation and purification of insert DNA
2. Isolation of vector DNA
3. Construction of Recombinant DNA
4. Introduction of Recombinant DNA into host cell
5. Identification or selection of cell containing cloned genes.

1. **Isolation and purification of insert DNA:** The gene of interest or insert DNA can be isolated either from bacterial cells or from plant cells or from animal cells. The various steps involved in the isolation and purification of DNA of follows:
   • The bacterial cells are grown in nutrient both and for concentrated by centrifugation.
   • These cells were treated with lysozyme (digest the cell wall) followed by EDTA (digest the cell envelope and prevents degradation of cellular DNA) that release the cell lysate.
   • The cell lysate (DNA, RNA and Some proteins plus cell debris) is purified to obtain only DNA molecule.

Purification involves; lysate is treated with a protease enzyme such as protinase or protinase K which breaks the proteins and poly peptides. Then this extract is treated with phenol chloroform. The treat with RNase that degrades RNA which is collected by centrifugation. The remaining aqueous layer is treated with absolute alcohol in presence of Sodium at a low temperature due to which DNA gets precipitated and is collected by centrifugation.

The purity of the sample is tested using absorbance at 260 nm and 280 nm. If the ratio is 1.8 it is taken as pure (< 1.8 indicates contamination with protein or phenol, > 1.8 indicates contamination of RNA)

2. **Isolation of Vector DNA**
   - To separate plasmid DNA from chromosomal DNA the method involves isopycnic centrifugation clear extract, in a solution of CsCl contacting Ethidium Bromide.
   - Ethidium Bromide binds by intercalating between DNA base pairs in doing so, cause the DNA to unwind.
   - A covalently closed circular DNA (CCC DNA) such as plasmid has no free ends and can only unwind to a limited extent, these limiting the amount of Ethidium Bromide bound. A linear DNA molecule, which as chromosomal DNA has no such topological barriers and can therefore find more ethidium bromide molecules.
   - Because as the density of the ethidium bromide DNA complex decreases as more ethidium bromide is bound.
   - As more ethidium bromide can be bound to linear molecules than a covalent circle, the plasmid has a higher density at saturating levels of ethidium bromide. Thus plasmid can be separated from linear chromosomal DNA.

3. **Construction of Recombinant DNA Invitro:** The next step in gene cloning is to insert the DNA sequence of interest into the plasmid to produce the Recombinant DNA. The technique of recombinant DNA in invitro involves the following steps:
   The insert DNA and plasmid DNA are cut with the restriction enzymes. Same type of rest enzymes are used for both DNase.
   The rest enzyme may give either sticky (or) cohesive ends or blunt ends. But in gene cloning it is desirable to have sticky ends. If blunt ended molecules are produced they can be converted to sticky ends by introducing either "linkers" or Adaptors "or by Homopolymer tailing. The sticky ends of DNA of interest and plasmid are joined by using DNA ligase and the process is called "DNA Ligation"

4. **Introduction of Recombinant DNA into host cells:**
   Introduction of recombinant DNA into host cells is called "Transformation". This is done with a view to produce innumersable amount of copies of insert

DNA. E.coli cells are used generally as host cells. The DNA can be introduced into cells by any one of the following methods;

> ➤ Use of viral vectors
> ➤ Microinjection
> ➤ Calcium phosphate mediated DNA uptake
> ➤ Liposome mediated gene transfer
> ➤ Electrophoresis

5. **Identification or selection of cells containing cloned genes:** After transformation the recombinant DNA gets multiplies along with the multiplication of the host cells. The next step in gene cloning, is to identify these transformed cells which actually easy the gene of interest. In bacteria, the cells carrying the recombinant plasmids are identified by anyone of the following methods:

> ➤ Selection through complementation of nutritional defects.
> ➤ Selection based on antibiotic resistance
> ➤ Selection through assay of biological activity
> ➤ Selection by immune chemical methods
> ➤ Selection through colony hybridization etc.

Strategies of cloning: The strategies or methods of gene cloning fall into 3 types. They are; 1) Shot gun method 2) cDNA cloning 3) cloning by gene synthesis

These strategies mainly depend upon

> ➤ The nature of target DNA
> ➤ The availability of screening methods
> ➤ The selection scheme

Cloning may involve a specific fragment of DNA and An entire genome.

1. **Shot gun method:** Cloning of an entire genome of an organism is called shot gun cloning. This involves the following steps:

> ➤ An entire genome is isolated
> ➤ The genome is cut into many small pieces at random either by mechanical shearing or by using rest enzymes.
> ➤ Plasmids of E.Coli are opened with the same rest enzyme and the DNA fragments are ligated into them. The recombinant DNA

102

plasmids are introduced into E.Coli to facilitate replication of DNA. These E.Coli cells are said to transformed.

➤ The transformed E.Coli is cultured to produce a large no of colonies each carrying a different piece of DNA. This collection of colonies constitutes a Genebank or Gene Library or Genomic Library.

Full length cDNA Cloning:
cDNA using plasmid vector and Cloning by Gene synthesis:
This technique involves the artificial synthesis of the desired DNA sequence or gene invitro by either of this way Khorana.

➤ Phosphodiester approach
➤ Phosphotriester approach
➤ Phosphate triester approach
➤ Enzymatic synthesis of DNA.

Then this is directly cloned into plasmid and then transformed into E.Coli.

Chapter 15
KARYOTYPING

The process of arrangement of chromosomes in a sequence according to the structure and size is called karyotyping.

Karyotyping is a technique that is used for identification of chromosome.

Culture of chromosome and preparation:

In general the methods of preparation chromosomes are varied.

- Chromosome s can be obtained from somatic cells by culturing them.
- One can undertake either short-term (or) long-term culture depending upon the cells used.
- Under long term culture one can use fibroblasts (or) amniotic fluid cells
- Chromosomes can also be observed directly (without culture) in tissue with high mitotic index like bone marrow (or) chorionic villous samples. The most common blood samples for fetal abnormalities are taken from the bone marrow.

Procedure:

Collection of blood: 1 to 5ml blood withdrawn from a vein heperinized and treated with phytohaemogglutanine (PHA)

Culture Medium:

- Prepare sterile culture bottle of 100ml, is medicated and provided with screw gap and then take 20ml of culture medium T.C.199
- Use 10ml pipette, flame it top to bottom and then the open end and closed end.

- Remove serum blood sample and transfer top layer of sediment along with some RBC.
- Gently shake the cell to from cell suspension.
- Transfer 10ml culture medium with suspended cells to second culture bottle.
- Incubate for at 37^0c after treatment with streptomycin and penicillin for mitosis.
- Add 0.5 of colchicine after 78hours and again after 30mins.
  Function of colchicine: Colchicine arrest centrifugation at metaphase by formation of a microtubule achromatic spindle at metaphase.

Centrifuge:

After 72hours take 10ml cell suspension from the culture bottle and it is transferred into centrifuged tube and the centrifuge for 10min (800-1000 RPM).

- Hypotonic solution (K^+, CL^-) is added and incubated for10min at 37^0C.

Function: allows celling, so that the cells are broken easily. Then the cells are dropped from height into the hypotonic solution then mix and add fixatives (glacial acetic acid in a ratio of 1:3) to the palate of cells. Gently shacked leading to the formation of cell suspension. Add a drop of the cell suspension on chemically cleaned slide from a certain height and stain with Giemsa stain under the microscope, this is followed by high power photograph. The individual chromosome has been cut out and arranged in decreasing order of size and number 1-22 with 2sex chromosome indicated separately. The resulting arrangement of the karyotype is called as karyotyping.

Karyotype:

Precise identification of individual chromosomes is now made possible by noting the banding pattern after applying the following stains.

Q-banding

G-banding

Classification of human chromosomes:

At a conference of geneticists held in "Denver in 1960" human chromosomes are classified into 7 groups

1. Group-A: 1-3 pairs (long metacentric) - long
2. Group-B: 4-5 pairs (sub metacentric centromere) - medium long
3. Group-C: 6-12 pairs (sub metacentric) - medium
4. Group-D: 13-15 pairs (acrocentric) - sub medium
5. Group-E: 16-18 pairs (sub metacentric) - small size
6. Group-F: 19-20 pairs (metacentric) - little small size
7. Group-G: 21-22 pairs acrocentric chromosome XY satellite body is present

Autosomal abnormalities (or) chromosomal disorders:

Cri-du chat syndrome: (karyotype- 5p)

Paou's syndrome: (karyotype – trisome 13)

Edward's syndrome: karyotype-trisome 18

<u>Down syndrome:</u> (London Down was discovered 1866)

Down's syndrome affected individual show round face with epicanthic fold (hence called Mongolism Down's.

Risk Down's (21 translocation)

Genotype: 47 XXX + 21

47 XXY +21

Phenotype: female

Clinical features:

- Mouth constantly opening
- Mental retardation
- Nose oblique, with short nose
- Flat nasal bridge

- Small ears (mal forming)
- Congenital heart disease (CHD)
- Hands shorter and broad their may be similar increase

Klinefelter's syndrome: (Harry Klinefelter's in 1942)

Genotype: 47XXY (trisome)

Phenotype: Male

Clinical features:

- Weak facial hair growth
- They are toll in stature
- They are sterile male and mentally effected
- Male sex glands and hormone are poorly developed
- They show Gynaecomastia (Excess of breast)

Turner's syndrome: (Turner's in 1940)

Genotype: 45 X 0 (monosome)

Phenotype: female

Clinical features:

- They are sterile female
- Short structure
- No menstruation
- They are normal in intelligence
- Broad chest, poor nipple,
- Low sex hormones, and poor growth of gonads
- They have low set of ears

Fragile X syndrome:

- This is so named because in squash preparation of cultured material X chromosome readily fractures at a particular site.
- The distal end of long arm of X chromosome shows a gap as a "fragile" site at the level of Xp 27.3
- This phenomena is caused by mutation involving on X chromosome of the female who acts as a carrier

Clinical features: mental retardation, big ears, and protrusion of chin, big hands and feet.

Chimaeras:

- So far we have seen what is a "mosaic" let us now consider another term "chimaera".
- Chimaera is an individual having 2 or more genetically different cell population derived from more than on zygote.
- Originally chimaera was named after a Greek histology and tail of dragon there are 2 types of chimaeras

  1. Dispermic chimaeras
  2. Blood group chimaeras

Chapter 16
POLYMERASE CHAIN REACTION (PCR)

The polymerase chain reaction results in the selective amplification of a chosen region of a DNA molecule. Developed in 1983 by **Kary Mullis,** PCR is now a common and often indispensable technique used in medical and biological research lab centre for a variety of applications. In 1993, **Mullis** was awarded Noble Prize in chemistry along with **Michael Smith** for his work on PCR. Upto 1985, cloning of genes of interest into prokaryotic and eukaryotic cell with the help of vector was considered to be essential tool for getting large identical copies of the gene in molecular biology.

- PCR is fast and easy when compared to cloning in recombinant DNA technology. Millions of copies of a DNA fragment can be obtained in a few hours by PCR.
- The double stranded DNA is denatured and the strands that are separated are allowed to anneal the primers (forward and reverse). Then the two strands are allowed to extend using dNTPs (deoxynucleotide triphosphate) generating new strands complimentary to the template strands. About 30-35 cycles of denaturing, annealing and extension are carried out in a thermo cycler. PCR can be used to amplify DNA sequences from any sources – Human, Animal, Bacteria, viral.

To amplify genomic DNA for selected sequence using appropriate primers E.g. To genotype the *Alu insertion / deletion polymorphism in angiotensin converting enzyme (ACE) gene.*

Components:

1. Template DNA
2. Oligonucleotide primers
3. Heat stable DNA polymerase obtained from thermus aquaticus.
4. Deoxyribonucleotide triphosphates

1. Template DNA

It is the DNA that contains the target sequence to be amplified; the DNA with sequence interest is isolated.

2. PRIMER: The specificity of PCR essential depends on primers. The following factors are important in closing effective primers.

- General length of primers is around 17-34 nucleotides.
- It should not have more complementary sequences in the target site.
- There should not be more than three types of nucleotides in primers.
- There should not be complementary between 2 primers.
- The GC content of about 50% is ideal.

3. ENZYME

Taq-DNA polymerase is the most commonly used enzyme. It binds to ssDNA and synthesizes new DNA strand complementary to the original strand.

4. Deoxynucleotide triphosphates

- These are 4 bases in DNA [A,G,T,C]
- These are substrates for DNA polymerase
- They act as building blocks to synthesize new DNA.

Amplification is usually carried out by the DNA polymerase I enzyme from **Thermus Aquaticus,** a Taq-polymerase, are Thermostable, meaning that they are resistant to denaturation by heat treatment.

Amplification by PCR

The PCR master mix for 10 samples as follows:

Distilled water: 49.5 µl

1 x PCR buffer: 10 µl

2.0 Mm $MgCl_2$: 8 µl

200 µMdNTPs: 2 µl

0.5 μM Primer (forward): 5 μl
0.5 μM Primer (reverse): 5 μl
0.5U Taq DNA polymerase: 0.5 μl

Add 10 μl of PCR mix to each DNA samples (50 ng – 100 ng) aliquot in 0.2ml PCR tube. The PCR amplification is carried out in the Thermo cycler following PCR conditions given below:

MECHANISM OF PCR:
The target DNA is amplified through repeated cycles of DNA synthesis. Stages operating at different temperatures

1. Initial denaturation: 94°C/5 min
2. Denaturation: 94°C / 5 sec
3. Annealing: 58°C/30 sec 30 cycles
4. Extension: 72°C/30 sec
5. Final extension: 72°C/3 min

The amplified products are run in 2% agarose gel for genotyping 7

DENATURATION
The reaction mixture is heated to a high temperature (usually 94^0C) that leads to separation of DNA strands. Time required for this is 0.5.

ANNEALING
The denatured DNA is then exposed to large quantities of primer. The reaction is brought down to 40^0C.The primers bind to the ssDNA on either side of target sequence to be amplified primer directs DNA polymerase enzyme to copy only the target DNA sequence.

EXTENSION
The reaction is heated to 74^0 C at which DNA polymerase enzyme is most active. it synthesizes the target DNA in presence of large number of free DNA bases [dNTP]

The Tm can be determined by experimentally but is usually calculated from the simple formula:

Tm (4x [G+C]) +(2+[A+T])^{0}C.

In which [G+C] is the number of G and C nucleotides in the primer sequence, and [A+T] is the number of A and T nucleotides.

Advantage of this procedure is small DNA is enough to amplify to billion copies.

Limitations

1. Applicable to short DNA fragment only
2. Flanking sequence should be known
3. Extremely sensitive, therefore amplifies foreign DNA also if the sample is contaminated.
4. Polymerase chain reaction; it is in vitro amplification of DNA
5. Can produce multiple copies of gene of interest few hours
6. Flanking sequence of gene of interest must be known

Clinical applications:

- The DNA of hair, single drop of blood or semen is amplified by PCR to solve medico legal problems in forensic medicine.
- Diagnosis of bacterial & viral diseases
- Diagnosis of genetic diseases like thalassemia, and cystic fibrosis etc.
- Cancer detection like Leukemia and lymphomas etc.
- Prenatal diagnosis of certain disease.
- For preparation of molecular markers (probes)
- For study of polymorphism

Quantitative PCR (Q-PCR): The Used to measure of quantity of a PCR product (commonly in the real-time). It Is quantitatively measures of starting amounts of DNA, cDNA or RNA. Q-PCR is commonly used to determine whether a DNA sequence is present in a sample and the number of its copies in the sample. *Quantitative real-time PCR* has a high degree of precision. QRT-PCR methods use fluorescent dyes, such as Sybr Green, Eva Green or fluorophore-containing of DNA probes, such as TaqMan, to esti*mate* the amount of amplified to the product in real time. This is also better sometimes abbreviated to a RT-PCR (*Real Time* PCR) or RQ-PCR. QRT-PCR or RTQ-PCR are more appropriate contractions, since this RT-PCR is commonly refers to reverse transcription PCR.

Figure 16.1 Real Time PCR

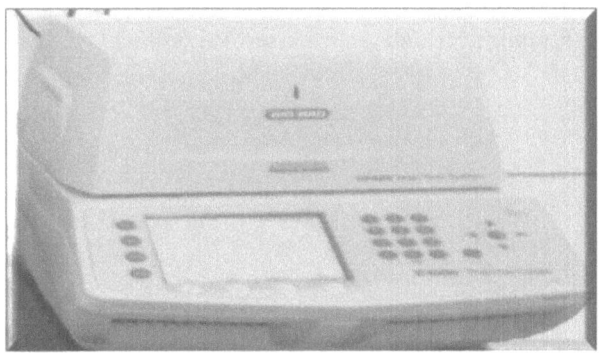

AFLP PCR

AFLP PCR **Background**

Amplified Fragment Length Polymorphism PCR, also called AFLP PCR was originally described by Zabeau et al., 1993.

AFLP is composed of 3 steps:

1-A) Cellular DNA is digested with one or more restriction enzymes. Typically this involves a combination of two restriction enzymes: a 4 base cutter (MseI) and a 6 base cutter (EcoRI).

1-B) Ligation of linkers (restriction half-site specific adaptors) to all restriction fragments.

2) Pre-selective PCR is performed using primers which match the linkers and restriction site specific sequences.

3) Electrophoretic separation and amplicons on a gel matrix, followed by visualization of the band pattern. The aim of this tool is to perform a theoretical AFLP-PCR experiment by using the same principles, and to suggest the adaptors and primers needed in the experiment.

Applications of AFLP PCR
AFLP is a highly sensitive PCR-based method for detecting polymorphisms in DNA. AFLP can be also used for genotyping individuals for a large number of loci using a minimal number of PCR reactions.

In Situ PCR

In Situ PCR (ISH) is a polymerase chain reaction that actually takes place inside the cell on a slide. *In situ* PCR amplification can be performed on fixed tissue or cells.

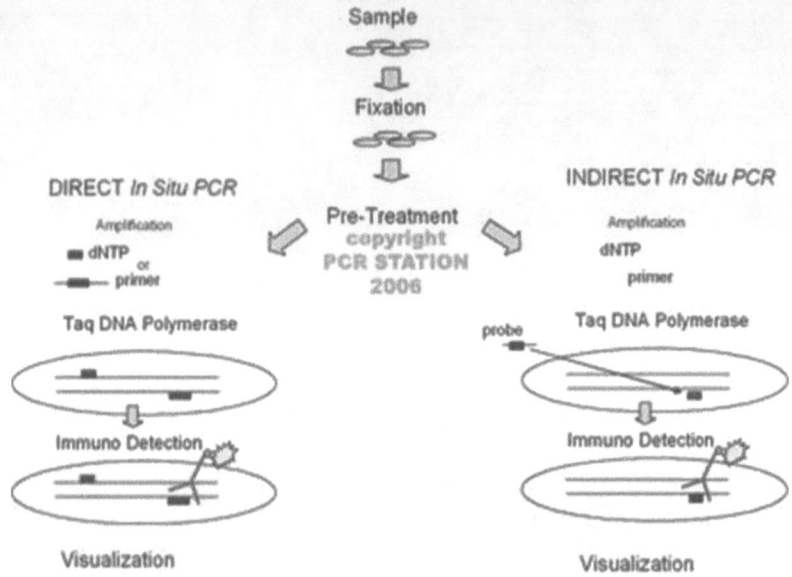

In Situ PCR

During the initiation and progression of disease, minute quantities of a product in small populations of cells or tissues may be vital for the pathogenesis of the disease.

In many slowly-evolving diseases which require months or even years to manifest themselves clinically, it has been shown that the majority of the affected cell population is in a transcriptionally inactive state, and at a level of one gene per host cell.

Nucleic acid hybridization methods and the polymerase chain reaction (PCR) have both been employed to examine the expression and detection of such affected genes during pathogenesis. While both these techniques are quite useful, the disadvantage of these techniques is that they are essentially conducting cell expression and population studies. Nucleic acids are isolated from a population of cells which contains either a sufficient number of molecules to detect directly by standard hybridization techniques, or, when a subpopulation contains as little as a single copy of nucleic acid, that molecule amplified by the PCR, and detected after amplification.

In situ hybridization (ISH) applies the methodology of the nucleic acid hybridization technique to the cellular level. Combining cytochemistry and immunocytochemistry, In Situ PCR allows the identification of cellular markers to be identified and further permits the localization of two cell specific sequences within cell populations, such as tissues and blood samples.

In Situ PCR is limited to the detection of non-genomic material such as RNA, genes or genomes, as the detection limit in most conditions is several copies of the target nucleic acid per cell. Therefore, due to copy number limitations, hybridization of RNA is more sensitive than DNA detection.

Factors affecting In Situ PCR sensitivity include:

1. The strangeness of the target molecule
2. The lack of a complementary sequence proximal to the target sequences

Reverse transcriptase-catalyzed *in situ* transcription has even been used to detect RNAs which occur at relatively high copy number.

REVERSE TRANSCRIPTASE-PCR

The reverse transcriptase-polymerase chain reaction involves the conversion of mRNA of a particular gene of interest present in the total RNA into cDNA and then amplifies a specific region of the cDNA. The enzyme reverse transcriptase catalyzes the conversion of mRNA into cDNA. This enzyme is isolated from retroviruses such as murine Maloney leukemia virus (MMLV) and avian myeloblastosis virus (AMV). It can also be synthesized using recombinant DNA technology. This technique is mainly used to assess the expression of genes. Reverse transcriptase-PCR can be done using a single step kit in which the reverse transcription reaction and the amplification can be carried out in a single vial.

For amplifying DNA from RNA. Reverse transcriptasereverse transcribes RNA into cDNA, which is then amplified by PCR. Quantification is carried out by Real-Time PCR, a modification of the standard PCR technique in which synthesis of the product is measured overtime, as the PCR proceeds through its series of cycles. RT-PCR is widely used in expression profiling, to determine the expression of a gene or to identify the sequence of an RNA transcript, including transcription start and termination sites. If the genomic DNA sequence of a gene is known,

RT-PCR can be used to map the location of exonsand introns in the gene. The 5' end of a gene (corresponding to the transcription start site) is typically identified by RACE-PCR (*Rapid Amplification of cDNA Ends*).

PRINCIPLE: RT-PCR selectively amplifies the first strand of cDNA that has been synthesized in vitro from mRNA templates by reverse transcription. The cDNA is first denatured by heating in the presence of a large molar excess of the two oligonucleotide primers and the four dNTPs. The reaction mixture is then cooled to temperature that allows the oligonucleotide primers to anneal to their target sequences, after which the annealed primers are extended with DNA polymerases. The cycle of denaturation, annealing and DNA synthesis is then repeated many times.

TWO STEP RT-PCR PROTOCOL

FIRST-STRAND cDNA SYNTHESIS PROTOCOL COMPONENTS OF THE KIT (INVITROGEN):
Superscript TM III RT (200U/μl)
5X First-strand buffer 250m M Tris-Hcl (pH 8.3 at room temperature), 375nM KCl, 15mM MgCl2
0.1m DTT

UNIT DEFINITION
One unit incorporates 1nmol of dTTP into acid – precipitately material in 10 min at 370C using poly (A). Oligo (dt) 25 as template primers.

STORAGE BUFFER
20mM Tris-HCl (pH7.5), 100mM NaCl,0.1mM EDTA,1mM DTT, 0.01%(v/v) NP-40, 50% (v/v) glycerol. (Store all components at -200C (non-frost-free). Thaw 5X first-strand Buffer and 0.1 M DTT at room temperature just prior to use and refreeze immediately.

FIRST –STRAND CDNA SYNTHESIS PROTOCOL
The following 20μl reaction volume can be used for 10 pg- 5μg of total RNA or 10 pg- 500ng of mRNA.

1. Add the following components to a nuclease free micro centrifuge tube:
   a. 1μl of Oligo(dT)20 (50μM) [200-500ng of Oligo(dT)12-18 or 50-250ng of random primers; or 2pmol of gene –specific primer]

    b.   10pg-5µg totalRNA or 10pg-500ng mRNA

    c.   1µl 10mM dNTP Mix (10mM each dATP,dGTP,dCTP and dTTP at neutral pH)

    d.   Sterile distilled water -13µl

    e.   Heat mixture to 650C for 5 min and incubate on ice for atleast 1 min.

2. Collect the contents of the tube by brief centrifugation and add:
   a. 4 µl 5X first-strand buffer
   b. 1 µl 0.1 M DTT
   c. 1 µlRNase out TM Recombinant RNase inhibitor (cat. No. 10777-019, 40 units/ µl)
   d. Note: When using less than 50 ng of starting RNA the addition of RNase OUTTM is essential.
   e. 1 µl of SuperscriptTMIII RT (200 units/ µl)

3. If generating cDNA longer than 5 kb at temperatures above 500C using a gene specific primer or oligo(dt)20, the amount of SuperscriptTMIII RT may be raised to 400 units (2µl) to increase yield.

4. Mix by pipetting gently up and down. If using random primers, incubate tube at 250C for 5 min.

5. Incubate at 500C for 30-60 min. Increase the reaction temperature to 550C for gene specific primer. Reaction temperature may also be increased to 550C for difficult templates or templates with high secondary structures.

6. Inactivate the reaction by heating at 700C for 15 min.

The cDNA can now be used as a template for amplification in PCR. However, amplification of some PCR targets (that > 1 kb) may require the removal of RNA complementary to the cDNA. To remove RNA complementary to the cDNA, add 1 µl (2 units) of E-coli RNase and incubate at 370C for 20 min. 22

STANDARD RT PROTOCOL – FIRST STRAND DNA SYNTHESIS

1. Oligodt (10µm) --5µl
2. dNTP (10µm)-- 1µl
3. RNA Template (1µg)   Varies
4. Sterile water   Varies

It was incubated at 65oC for 5 min and kept in ice for atleast 2 min, Centrifuge and collect the contents

1.   First strand buffer
2.   4µl DTT (0.1M)
3.   1µl Superscript III RT   0.2µl
4.   Total amount 20µl

Restriction Fragment Length Polymorphism (RFLP)
Mutations, variations, recombination's may bring about changes in genomic DNA sequences. These changes in DNA sequence may generate or abolish or after the position of recognition site for rest endonucleases. To find out these changes the technique applied is RFLP.

Procedure
First the genomic DNA's are isolated. They are digested with restriction enzymes and then electrophoresis. These were blotted on to a membrane and detected with radio labeled probe. Then polymorphism in hybridization pattern is revealed due to change in restriction site cleavage such variation is termed as restriction fragment length polymorphism.

PCR Reaction Mixture
PCR master mix for 10 samples
Distilled water: 220.125 µl
1 x PCR buffer: 37.5 µl
2.0 mMMgC12: 30.5µl
200 µMdNTPs: 7.5 µl
0.5 µM Primer (forward): 14.0 µl
0.5 µM Primer (reverse): 14.0 µl and 0.5U Taq DNA polymerase: 1.875 µl

Add 13 µl of PCR mix to each DNA samples (50 ng – 100 ng) aliquot in 0.2ml PCR tube.
The PCR amplification is carried out in the Thermocycler following the PCR conditions given below:

1.   Initial denaturation: 94°C/5 min
2.   Denaturation: 94°C / 45 sec
3.   Annealing: 64°C/30 sec 30 cycles
4.   Extension: 72°C/30 sec
5.   Final extension: 72°C/3 min

5µl of PCR amplified products are run in 1.5% agarose gel to check for amplification. 8

Application:

- It is very much useful in gene mapping. For the detection of genetic defects in Huntington's disease cystic fibrosis, sickle cell anemia etc.
- Indifferent strain identifications, and epidemiological typing.
- RFLP is also used in forensic medicine.
- RFLP is also used for evolutionary studies.
- To characterize germ plasma source.
- For cytogenetic studies are plants.

Restriction Digestion
The amplified products are digested with appropriate restriction enzymes

Reaction Mix for 10 samples

Distilled water: 87 µl
1 x Buffer: 10 µl
3 U Restriction Enzyme: 3 µl
Add 10 µl of the above mix to 10 µl of PCR product and incubate it at 65°C for 3 hours. After digestion is completed run the samples along with DNA marker in 2% agarose gel.

Interpretation
Based on the number of bands the samples with and without restriction site are identified and genotyped.

4. Random Amplified Polymorphic DNA (RAPD)

The Random Amplified Polymorphic DNA (RAPD) method is based on the PCR using short (usually 10 nucleotide) primers of arbitrary sequences. Polymorphism of amplified fragments are caused by: base substitutions or deletions in the priming sites, Insertions that render priming sites too distant to support amplification, or insertions or deletions that change the size of the amplified fragment. RAPD technique may be used to determine taxonomic identity, assess kinship relationships, analyze mixed genome samples, and create specific probes.

Aim: To detect the polymorphism of the given target gene using defamer primers.

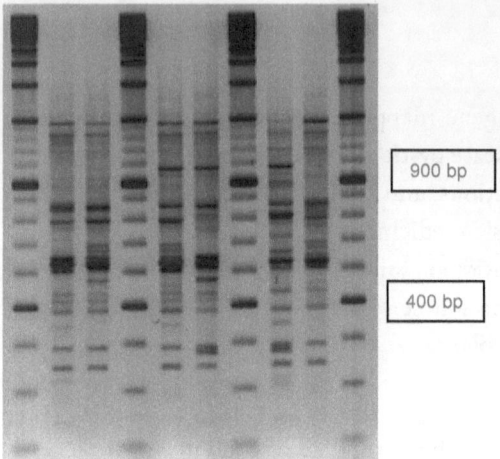

RAPD polymorphisms in the stoneroller fish (Campostomaanomalum) trapped in tributaries of the Great Miami River in Ohio. Each pair of samples is flanked by a lane containing DNA size standards; in these lanes, the smallest DNA fragment is 100 base pairs (bp), and each successively larger fragment increases in size by 100 bp. Fragments whose sizes are multiples of 500 bp are present in greater concentration and so yield darker bands.

Amplification by PCR

The PCR master mix for 1 samples as follows:

MilliQwater: 14.5μl
1 x PCR buffer: 2 μl
2.0 mMMgC12: 1 μl
200 μMdNTPs: 0.5 μl
0.5 μMPrimer: 0.5 μl
0.5U Taq DNA polymerase: 0.5 μl
Template DNA: 1 μl
Add 10 μl of PCR mix to each DNA samples (50 ng – 100 ng) a liquored in 0.2ml PCR tube. The PCR amplification is carried out in the Thermo cycler following PCR conditions given below:

    6. Initial denaturation: 94°C/5 min
    7. Denaturation: 94°C /1 min

8. Annealing: 36°C/1 min 34 cycles
9. Extension: 72°C/2 min
10. Final extension: 72°C/7 min

The amplified products are run in 2% agarose gel for detecting polymorphism 10

SDS-Polyacrylamide Gel Electrophoresis (PAGE)

Principle

Electrophoresis is the study of the movement of charged molecules in an electric field. The generally used support medium is cellulose or thin gels made up of either polyacrylamide or agarose. Cellulose is used as support medium for low molecular weight biochemical such as amino acid and carbohydrates whereas agarose and Polyacrylamide gels are widely used for larger molecules like proteins. The general electrophoresis techniques cannot be used to measure the molecular weight of the biological molecules because the mobility of a substance in the gel is influenced by both charge and size. In order to overcome this, if the biological samples are treated so that they have a uniform charge, electrophoretic mobility then depends primarily on size. The molecular weight of protein maybe estimated if they are subjected to electrophoresis in the presence of a detergent sodium dodecyl sulfate (SDS) and a reducing agent mercaptoethanol (ME).

SDS disrupts the secondary, tertiary and quaternary structure of the protein to produce a linear polypeptide chain coated with negatively charged SDS molecules. 1.4grams of SDS binds per gram of protein. Mercaptoethanol assists the protein denaturation by reducing all disulfide bonds.

SDS-Polyacrylamide Gel Electrophoresis (PAGE)

Polyacrylamide gels are prepared by the free radical polymerization of acrylamide and the cross linking agent N N' methylene bis acrylamide

Acrylamide + N N' methylene bis acrylamide

Chemical Ammonium per sulfate (catalyst)
Polymerization +
TEMED (N, N N' N' tetramethylethylenediamine)
Polyacrylamide

Reagents Preparation

1. Acrylamide Solution:
9g Acrylamide
300 mg Bisacrylamide
Dissolved in 30ml of Distilled water and incubated overnight in brown bottle using magnetic stirrer.

2. Running Buffer (Tank Buffer):
14.4 g of Glycine
3.0 g of Trisbase
1.0 g of SDS
Dissolved in 1 litre of Distilled water

3. 10% Sodium do decylsulfate:0.1 g in 1 ml water
4. 10% Ammonium per sulphate:0.1 g in 1 ml water
5. Stacking Buffer (1 M):

3.63 g Tris in 20 ml water.
Adjust the pH to **6.8** with 0.1 N HCL and made the total volume to 30 ml.

6. Resolving Buffer (1.5 M):

9.06 g Tris in 30 ml water.
Adjust the pH to **8.8** with 0.1 N HCL and made the total volume to 50 ml.

7. Sample Buffer:

392 mg Trisbase
600 mg SDS
5.2 ml Glycerol
0.6 ml β Mercaptoethanol
30 mg Bromophenol blue
Adjust the pH to **6.8** using 0.1 N HCL and Made upto 20 ml water

Procedure:

1. Assembling the glass plate (Demonstration)

Note:

Gloves should be worn at all times while performing SDS-PAGE.

To ensure proper alignment and casting, the glass plates, spacers, combs and casting stand gaskets must be clean and dry. The glass plates should be cleaned with 70% ethanol.

1. Assemble the glass plate on a clean surface. Lay the longer glass plate down first, then place 2 spacers of equal thickness along the rectangular plate. Next place the shorter glass plate on top of the spacers so that the bottom ends of the spacers and glass plates are aligned.
2. Loosen the 4 screws on the clamp assembly and stand it up so that the screws are facing away from you. Firmly grasp the glass plate sandwich with the longer plate facing away from you, and gently slide it into the clamp assembly. Tighten the top 2 screws of the clamp assembly.
3. Place the clamp assembly into the alignment slot of the casting stand so that the clamp screws face away from you. Loosen the top 2 screws to allow the plates and spacers to sit firmly against the casting stand base. Gently tighten all the screws.
4. Pull the completed sandwich from the alignment slot. Check that the plates and spacers are aligned. If not, realign the sandwich as in steps 1-3. Before transferring the clamp assembly to the casting slot, recheck the alignment of the spacers. Do this by inverting the gel sandwich and looking at the surface of the 2 glass plates and the spacer. Make sure that they are aligned.
5. Transfer the clamp assembly to one of the casting slots in the casting stand. If 2 gels are to be prepared, place the clamp assembly on the other side of the alignment slot.
6. Press the acrylic pressure plate bottom, so that the glass plates rest on the rubber gasket. Snap the acrylic plate underneath the overhang of the casting slot. Do not push the glass plates or spacers because this could break the glass plate.

2. Casting the gels (Demonstration)

Prepare 10% resolving/separating gel and 5% stacking gel (Table 1)

1. Prepare the **separating gel monomer** solution by combining all reagents except ammonium persulfate (APS) and TEMED. Deaerates and mixes the solution after adding each reagent by swirling the container gently.
2. Place a comb completely into the assembled gel sandwich. With a marker pen, place a mark on the glass plate 1 cm below the teeth of the comb. This will be the level to which the separating gel is poured. Remove the comb.
3. Add APS and TEMED to the monomer solution and mix well by swirling gently. Pipette the solution to the mark.
4. Immediately overlay the monomer solution with 1 ml of water. Use a steady, even rate of delivery to prevent mixing with the gel.
5. Allow the gel to polymerize for 10 minutes. Pour the water overlaying the gel and drain the excess water with strips of filter paper.
6. Prepare the **stacking gel** monomer solution. Combine all reagents except APS and TEMED. Deaerate and mix the solution by swirling gently.
7. Place a comb in the gel sandwich.
8. Allow the gel to polymerize for 10 minutes.
9. Remove the comb.
10. Gel is placed in the buffer chamber and running gel buffer is added into the chamber 3.

Preparation of Sample:

While the stacking gel is polymerizing, prepare the samples in appropriate volume of 1X SDS gel- loading buffer and heat them to 100 °C for 3 minutes to denature the proteins.

Load upto 15 µl of each of the samples in a predetermined order in to the bottom of the wells.

Attach the electrophoresis apparatus to an electric power supply (The positive electrode should be connected to the bottom buffer reservoir). Apply the voltage of 50V/cm to the gel. After the dye front has moved into the resolving gel, increase the voltage to 100V/cm and run the gel until the bromophenol blue reaches the bottom of the resolving gel (3 hr). Then turn off the power supply.

Remove the glass plates from the electrophoresis apparatus and place them on a paper towel. Use an extra gel spacer to carefully pry the plates apart. Mark the orientation of the gel by cutting a corner from the bottom of the gel that is closest to the left most well (Do not cut the corner from the gels).

Then the gel can be fixed, stained with Coomassie Brilliant Blue or Silver salts.

4. Preparation of Staining Solution

1. Coomassie Brilliant Blue

Staining Solution

Coomassive blue R250 – 1.2 g (0.2%) [Dissolve in methanol]
Methanol 500 ml (50%), Glacial Acetic acid 200 ml (7%) and Distilled water 500 ml

Distaining Solution

Methanol 300 ml (50%),Glacial Acetic acid 100 ml (7%) and Distilled water 1 liter

2. Silver Staining

Reagent Preparation

MFA (100 ml)

50 ml Methanol,50 µl formaldehyde, 12 ml Acetic acid and 38 ml Distilled water

50 ml ethanol and 50 ml Distilled water

Silver Nitrite

200 mg $AgNO_3$
72 µl formaldehyde
100 ml water

Sodium Thiosulphate (STS)

Stock – 100 mg STS / 10 ml Distilled water
2ml Stock STS and 98 ml water

Sodium Carbonate

6 g Sodium carbonate
400 µl Stock STS
50 µl formaldehyde and Make upto 100 ml with water

Protocol

1. Add MFA over the Gels for (1hour) in shaker
2. Discard MFA
3. Add 50 % Ethanol, wash 20 min for 3 times
4. Add STS for 3 times, 1 min each
5. Water wash
6. Add Ag NO3 (8 to 10 min)
7. Water wash for 1 min
8. Add Sodium Carbonate (Shake well until protein bands are visible)
9. Add MFA for 1 min and keep it in shaker
10. Discard MFA and Store the gel in water

Glossary

1. **Acentric: The** Acentric fragment of the chromosome with two centromeres will break unevenly during mitosis, resulting in one daughter chromosome lacking essential genes.

2. **Activator:** A DNA- binding protein that regulates one or more genes by increasing the rate of transcription.

3. **Adenine:** Adenine is one of the two purine nucleobases used in forming nucleotides of the nucleic asids DNA and RNA. It is a purine component of nucleic acids and nucleotides. Adenine always forms complementary base-paring with thymine.

4. **Adenosine: A purine nucleoside which is found endogenously, composed of a molecule of adenine** base attached to a ribose sugar. It is a nitrogen-containing compound.

5. **Adenosine phosphates:** A group of organic phosphates including adenosine monophosphate (AMP), adenosine diphosphate (ADP) and adenosine triphosphate (ATP). They function nin phosphate transfer in the cell, particularly in the transfer of the high-energy phosphate bonds of ADP and ATP. ATP is the most directly utilized source of energy of the cell.

6. **Adenylation**: also known as adenylylation or AMPylation, is the process of attaching an AMP molecule to a protein side chain by covalent bonding.

7. **Adenyl cyclase**: An enzyme which catalyzes the formation of cyclic AMP from ATP by the removal of pyrophosphate.

8. **A Form**: A duplex DNA structure with right- handed twisting in which the planes of the base pairs are tilled about 70^0 with respect to the helix axis.

9. **Alleles:** The various forms of a gene are called Alleles. For example, blue colour and black colour of eye are two alleles of the eye colour.

10. **α- amantin:** Toxin that inhibits the eukaryotic RNA polymerases to different extents and thus useful in characterizing them.

11. **Aminoacyl-transfer RNA (aa-tRNA)**: The molecule produced when an amino acid is activated into its amino-acyl form and attached to its specific

transfer – RNA molecule, the whole process being catalyzed by a specific aminoacyl tRNA synthatase enzyme.

12. **Amplification:** A increase in the number of copies of a specific DNA fragments; can be in vivo or in vitro

13. **Amitosis:** Direct division of nucleolus into two, without differentiation of chromosomes of chromosomes and formation of spindle etc.

14. **Amphimixis:** Union of nuclear material from male and female gametes during the process of fertilization.

15. **Anaphase:** The stage of mitosis when sister chromatids of each chromosome separate and move to opposite poles of the spindle.

16. **Aneuploids:** Having non-balanced number of chromosmes, and not an exact multiple of haploid set.

17. **Anticodon:** Three adjacent nucleotides in transfer RNA that bind to a codon of three adjacent nucleotide is messenger RNA during protein synthesis.

18. **Antiparallel:** Describing two linear polymer that are opposite in polarity or orientation.

19. **ARS**: Autonomously replicating sequence; the origin of replication in yeast.

20. **A-Site:** The binding site on a ribosome that holds the tRNA carrying the next amino acid to be added to a growing polypeptide chain.

21. **ATP**: Most important high energy molecules, ie. Energy currency of the cell. Synthesized by oxidative phosphorylation, and substance level phosphorylation.

22. **ATPase**: An enzyme that hydrolase ATP to yield ADP and phosphate.

23. **ATP synthetase**: An enzyme complex that forms ATP from ADP and phosphate.

24. **Autoradiography**: The detection of radioactive molecules (eg, DNA, RNA, protein) by visualization of their effects on photographic or x-ray film.

25. **Autosome:** chromosomes other than the sex chromosomes. Theys are similar in both males and females.

26. **Bacteriophage**: The virus that infect the bacterium, also termed as bacterial virus.

27. **B Form**: The most common form of duplex DNA, containing a right-handed helix and about 10 (10.5 exactly) base pairs per turn of the helix axis.

28. **Back-Mutation:** A mutation that causes a mutant gene to regain its wild-type base sequence.

29. **Base Analog:** A compound, usually a purine or a pyrimidine, that differs some what from a normal nucleic acid base.

30. **Base pair (bp)**: Two nucleotides in a DNA or an RNA molecule that are paired by hydrogen bonds, for example, G pairs with C, and A pairs with T or U.

31. **Base stacking**: The close packing of the planes of base pairs, commonly found in DNA and RNA structures.

32. **Base sequence:** The order of base nucleotide bases in a DNA molecule

33. **B-DNA**: The naturally-occurring form of DNA duplexes in vivo, that is the same as the model proposed by Watson and Crick in 1953.

34. **Bidirectional Replication**: Replication in both directions away from the origin, as opposed to replication in one direction only (unidirectional replication)

35. **Blocks**: Blocks uses multiply aligned ungapped segments corresponding to the most highly conserved regions or proteins. Block searcher, Get Blocks and Block Maker are aids to detection and verification of protein sequence homology. They compare a protein or DNA sequence to a database of protein blocks, retrieve blocks, and create new blocks, respectively.

36. **Blunt-ended DNA**: Two strands of a DNA duplex having ends that are flush with each other.

37. **Bond**: A force holding atoms together in a chemical compound; the principal types of bond are covalent, ionic, and hydrogen.

38. **Branch Migration:** Movement of the branch point in branched DNA formed from two DNA molecules with identical sequences.

39. **Cancer**: The cells continue to divide and give rise to a malignant tumour. These cells can also invade other tissues and tumours. These cells can also invade other tissues and tumours can arise inh new locations.

40. **5' Cap**: 7-methyl-guanosine structure added to the beginning of eukaryotic mRNAs.

41. **Centimorgan (cM):** A unit of measure of recombination frequency. One centimorgan is equal to a 1% chance that a marker at one genetic locus will be separated from a marker at a second locus due to crossing over in a single generation. In human beings, 1 centimorgan is equivalent, on average, to 1 million base pairs.

42. **Central dogma of molecular genetics**: The hypothesis (based on Weismannism) that genetically information flows only in one direction, from DNA to RNA to protein, and not in the opposite direction; refers to how genes work to make proteins; each protein-coding gene is transcribed

into a molecule of mRNA, which is translated into a sequence of amino acids that comprise a polypeptide (i.e., a protein).

43. **Centromere: The region of a chromosome to which spindle fibre attaches.**

44. **cDNA**: A single-stranded DNA molecule that is complementary to an mRNA molecule and is synthesized from it by the action of reverse transcriptase.

45. **Chemical bond**: The force that holds atoms together in molecules.

46. **Chemotherapy**: The use of chemical substances to combat disease caused by microorganisms; the term is often extended to include cancer treatment by chemicals.

47. **Chimeric molecule**: A molecule3 (eg, DNA, RNA, protein) containing sequences derived from two different species.

48. **Chimeric DNA:** A recombinant DNA containing genes from two different species.

49. **Chloramphenicol (CAP):** A bacteriostatic antibiotic produced by the ascomycetous fungus, Streptomycin; inhibits protein synthesis in a variety of organisms.

50. **Chromatin:** Deep stained part of the nuclear reticulum mostly of DNA, which condenses into chromosome during cell division.

51. **Chromomere:** A small deeply stained particle or granule in the chromosome, visible in the prophase of meiosis.

52. **Chromonemata:** The chromatin treads visible within the chromosome in the metaphase and anaphase stages of cell division.

53. **Chromosome:** The self-replicating genetic structures of cells containing the cellular DNA that bears in its nucleotide sequence the linear array of genes. In Prokaryotes, chromosomal DNA is circular, and the entire genome is carried on one chromosome. Eukaryotic genomes consist of a number of chromosomes whose DNA is associated with different kinds of proteins.

54. **Chromosomal Aberration:** Includes modifications or changes in the chromosomes. It may be loss or gain of a particular block of genes, rearrangement of a block of genes or loss gain of a chromosome, a pair of chromosomes or a complete set of chromosomes.

55. **Chromosomal Complement:** The group of chromosome derived from a particular nucleus. It usually comprises of one set in gametes (haploid) and two sets in a zygote.(diploid)

56. **Chromosome Puff:** A swollen region of a gaint chromosome; the swelling reflects a high degree of transcription activity.

57. **Cistron:** A unit of function, i.e, segment of DNA that determines a single polypeptide chain.

58. **Clone:** A carbon copy of the parent. A group of cells that are derived by mitotic divisions from a single ancestral cell.

59. **Cloning vector:** DNA molecule originating from a virus, a plasmid, or the cell of a higher organism into which another DNA fragment of appropriate size can be integrated without loss of the vector's capacity for self-replication; vectors introduce foreign DNA into host cells, where it can be reproduced in large quantities. Examples are plasmids, cosmids, and yeast artificial chromosomes; vectors are often recombinant molecules containing DNA sequences from several sources.

60. **ClustalW:** It is popular software for multiple sequence alignment. It can be used on either DNA or proteins. The output of ClustalW is a multiple alignment, shown graphically, and it can even construct phylogenetic trees according to the alignment. ClustalW creates alignments in a format called GCG. However, most alignment software and viewers uses another format, the Fasta format. The program tofasta converts files from GCG fromat to fasta format.

61. **Codon:** Triplet (group of three) of bases on mRNA that specify a perticular amino acid in protien synthesis.

62. **Colony hybridizatio:** It is a technique for using in situ hybridization to identify bacteria carrying chimeric vector whose inserted DNA is homologous with some particular sequence.

63. **Complementary:** Having a molecular surface with chemical groups arranged to interact specially with chemical groups on another molecule.

64. **Complementary Base sequence:** For a given sequence of nucleic acids, the nucleic acids that are related to them by the rules of base pairing.

65. **Complementary DNA (cDNA):** A DNA used in DNA cloning, usually made by reverse transcriptase; complementary to a given mRNA.

66. **Composite Transposon:** A DNA fragment having a central region flanked on each side by insertion sequence, either or both of which may enable the entire element to transpose.

67. **Consensus sequence:** A most typical form of a sequence that occurs with minor variations in a group of related DNA, RNA, or protein sequence. The consensus sequence show the nucleotide or amino acid most often

found at each position. The preservation of a consensus sequence implies that the sequence is functionally important.

68. **Conservative replication:** A form of DNA replication, where both strands of the parent DNA are transferred to one daughter molecule, whereas the other molecule has 2 newly, synthesized strands. Compare semiconservative replication, where one strand of the parent molecule ends up in each of the progeny molecule.

69. **Cointegrate:** An intermediate in the migration of certain DNA transposons which the donor DNA and target DNA are covalently attached.

70. **Controlling elements:** Transposable units originally identified solely by their genetic properties.

71. **Coordinate Regulation:** The common control of a group of genes.

72. **Cooperative Binding:** A situation in which the binding of one ligand to a macromolecule favors the binding of another. For example, DNA cooperatively binds histone molecules, and hemoglobin cooperatively binds oxygen molecule.

73. **Copy number variation (CNV):** Change in the copy number of specific genomic regions of DNA between two or more individuals. CNVs can be as large as $(10)6$ bp of DNA and include deletions or insertions.

74. **Cosmid:** A plasmid into which the DNA sequences from bacteriophage lambda that are necessary for the packaging of DNA (co sites) have been inserted; this permits the plasmid DNA to be packaged in vitro.

75. **Cot Curve:** A curve that indicates the rate of DNA-DNA annealing as a function of DNA concentration and time.

76. **Covalent bond:** co^{-L} = together + valare^{L} = to be strong): A stable chemical bond formed by the sharing of one or more pairs of electrons among the atoms in a molecule.

77. **Cyclic AMP, cAMP:** A second messenger within cells that are generated from ATP in response to hormonal stimulation of cell-surface receptors; cAMP acts as a signaling molecule by activating A-kinase; it is hydrolyzed to AMP by phosphodiesterase.

78. **Cyclic Photophosphorylation:** ATP synthesis driven by cyclic electron flow through photosystem I.

79. **Cytidine:** A pyrimidine nucleoside found in DNA and RNA.

80. **Cytosine:** A pyrimidine base found in DNA and RNA.

81. **D Loop:** An extended loop of single-stranded DNA displaced from a duplex structure by an oligonucleotide

82. **Dalton:** A unit of mass equivalent to the mass of hydrogen atom (1.66 x 10-24g)

83. **Deambulum (contains the Genomes):** Viruses, Archaea, Bacteria, Fungi, Plant, Animals and Man.

84. **Degeneracy:** Degeneracy in the genetic code refers to the lack of an effect of many changes in the third base of the codon on the amino acid that is represented.

85. **Deletion Mutation:** A mutation resulting from the deletion of one or more nucleotides from a gene or chromosome.

86. **Deletion (DNA):** The absence of chromosome segment.

87. **De novo pathway:** Pathway for synthesis of a biomolecule, such as a nucleotide, from simple precursors, as distinct from a salvage pathway.

88. **Denaturation:** It is the conversion of DNA from the double stranded to the single stranded state. Separation of strands is accomplished by heating or treating with alkali.

89. **Deoxyribose:** A type of sugar which is an important structural unit of DNA.

90. **Deoxyribonucleic acid (DNA):** A nucleic acid found in chromosomes, which stores heredity in formation in code-like manner.

91. **Discontinuous replication:** It refers to the synthesis of DNA in short, Okazaki fragments that are later joined into a continuous strand.

92. **DNA Chimera:** A DNA containing genetic information derived from two different species.

93. **DNA Cloning:** The propagation of individual segment of DNA as clones.

94. **DNA fingerprint:** The use of highly variable regions of the DNA sequence to identify an individual.

95. **DNA library:** A Collection of cloned DNA fragment s, usually representing an entire genome present in an organism. Also called genomic DNA library.

96. **DNA Ligase:** An enzyme that can seal one DNA fragment with another DNA segment both having sticky ends. Ligase is the "molecular glue".

97. **DNA Looping:** The interaction of proteins bound at distant sites on a DNA molecule so that the intervening DNA forms a loop.

98. **DNA polymerase:** An enzyme responsible for linking free DNA nucleotides to form the complementary strand. It can polymerise the nucleotides only in 5'-3' direction.

99. **DNA Replicase System:** The entire complex of enzymes and specialized proteins required in biological DNA replication. DNA supercoiling: The

coiling of DNA upon itself, generally as a result of bending, underwinding, or overwinding of DNA helix.

100. **DNA sequencing:** Determination of the order of nucleotides in a DNA molecule.

101. **Double helix:** The natural coiled conformation of two complementary, antiparellel DNA chains.

102. **Double reciprocal plot:** A plot of $1/V0$ versus $1/(S)$, which allow a more accurate determination of V_{max} and K_m than a plot of V_0 versus (S); also called the Line Weaver Burk plot.

103. **Drosophila melanogaster:** A species of small dipterous fly, commonly called a fruit fly; extgensively used in genetical studies of development.

104. **Duplication:** Type of chromosome rearrangement in which a gene sequence occurs in excess of its normal amount in a chromosome.

105. **EDP (Eukaryotic Promoter Database):** An annotated non-redundant collection of eukaryotic POL II promoters, for which the transcription start site has been determined experimentally.

106. **Elongation Factor:** Protein factors uniquely required during the elongation phase of protein synthesis. Elongation factor G (EF-G) brings about the movement of the peptidyl tRNA from the A site to the P site of the ribosome.

107. **eMotif:** eMotif also known as identify, uses data from Blocks and Finger Print to generate consensus expressions from the conserved regions of sequence alignments. eMotif adopts a "fuzzy" algorithm which allows certain amino acid alterations. This allows eMotif to find homologous sequence that other programs can not find, but it results in a lot of noise. This trade-off shows why it is important to use multiple programs when searching for information.

108. **ENCODE Project:** Encyclopedia of DNA Elements Project; an effort of multiple laboratories throughout the world to provide a detailed, biochemically informative representation of the human genome using high throughout sequencing methods to identify and catalog the functional elements within a single restricted portion (-1%; 30,000,000 bp) of one human chromosome.

109. **Endonuclease:** An enzyme that cleaves internal bonds in DNA or RNA.

110. Energy charge: (a term coined by Daniet Atkinson in 1970): It is a quantity that indicates the state of a cell's energy reserves. It is equal to the cell's reserves of the free energy sources, ATP and ADP (taking into account that ADP stores less free energy than ATP) divided by the total supply of

ATP and its breakdown products, ADP and AMP. Thus, Energy charge = [ATP] + ½ [ADP]/[ATP] + [ADP] = [AMP].

111. **Energy charge:** The fractional degree to which the ATP/ADP/AMP system in filled with high energy phosphate groups.

112. **Enhancer:** A DNA sequence that can stimulate transcription at an appreciable distance from the site where it is located. It acts is either orientation an either upstream or downstream from the promoter. DNA sequences that facilitate the expression of a given gene may be located a few hundred, or even thousand, base pairs away from the gene.

113. **Epigenetic code:** The patients of modification of chromosomal DNA (ie, cytosine methylation) and nucleosomal histone posttranslational modifications. These changes in modification status can lead to dramatic alterations in gene expression. Notably though, the actual underlying DNA sequence involved does not change.

114. **Episome:** It is a plasmid able to integrate into bacterial DNA.

115. **Escherichia coli:** A common rod like bacterium normally found in the small intestine (colon) of humans and other mammals; the most well studied organism; widely used in biomedical research; also called E.coli.

116. **Eukaryotic cell:** A type of cell which possesses a well-defined nuclear membrane.

117. **Excinuclease:** The excision nuclease involved in nucleotide exchange repair of DNA.

118. **Excision-repair:** Systems remove a single stranded sequence of DNA containing damaged or mispaired bases and replace it in the duplex by synthesizing a sequence complementary to the remaining strand.

119. **Exon:** The sequence of a gene that is represented (expressed) as mRNA.

120. **Exonuclease:** An enzyme that cleaves nucleotides from either the 3' or 5' ends of DNA or RNA.

121. **Expression vector:** It is a cloning vector designed so that a coding sequence inserted at a particular site will be transcribed and translated into protein.

122. **FAD(Flavin Adenine Dinucleotide):** The coenzyme of some oxidation-reduction enzymes; it contains riboflavein

123. **Fingerprinting:** The use of RFLPs or repeat sequence DNA to establish a unique pattern of DNA fragments for an individual.

124. **FISH:** Fluorescence in situ hy7bidization, a method used to map the location of specific DNA sequences within fixed nuclei.

125. **Flavin-**Linked Dehydrogenases: Dehydrogenases requiring one of the riboflavin coenzymes, FMN or FAD.

126. **FlavinNucleotides:** Nucleotide coenzyme (FMN and FAD) containing riboflavin.

127. **FlyBase:** It is a comprehensive database for information on the genetic and molecular biology of Drosophila. It includes data from the Drosophila Genome projects and data curated from the literature.

128. **Footprinting:** DNA with protein bound is resistant to digestion by Dnase enzymes. When a sequencing reaction is performed using such DNA, a protected area, representing the "footprint" of the bound protein, will be detected because nucleases are unable to cleave the DNA directly bound by the protein.

129. **Frame Shift Mutation:** Insertion or deletion of genetic material that lead to a shift in the translation of the reading frame. The mutation usually leads to nonfunctional proteins.

130. **Free energy (G):** The component of the total energy of a system that can do work at constant temperature and pressure and defined by the equation, $G = H - TS$, where H is the heat content (enthalpy), T the thermodynamic temperature, and S the entropy; takes into account changes in both energy and entropy.

131. **Furanose:** A sugar that contains a five-membered ring as a result of intramolecular hemiacetal formation. A simple sugar containing the five membered furan ring.

132. **G 1 Phase:** That period of the cell cycle in which preparations are being made for chromosome duplication, which takes place in the S phase.

133. **G 2 Phase:** That period of the cell cycle between S phase and mitosis (Mphase)

134. **Gap:** Absence of one or more nucleotides in one strand of the duplex DNA.

135. **Gene:** The basic unit of heredity located on a chromosome. It is equivalent to the 'factor' of Mendel. These words are units of information from one generation to another.

136. **Gene amplification:** A process in which many copies are made of some genes at one time, while other genes are not replicated. The replicated genes enable enhanced manufacture of product in a short time

137. **Gene bank:** (1). A collection of clones containing all the genes of a particular organism, such as Escherichia coli. (2). A collection of many lines of a particular crop plant, used as a genetic resource blue plant breeders.

138. **Gene Cards:** It is a database of human genes, their products and their involvements in disease.

139. **Gene cloning:** The technique of genetic engineering in which specific genes are excised from host DNA, inserted into a vector plasmid and introduced into a host cell, which then divides to produce many copies (clones) of the transferred gene.

140. **Gene dosage:** It is the relationship between nucleotide sequence in nucleic acids and amino acid sequence in protein.

141. **Gene expression:** Transcription and, in the case of proteins, translation to yield the product of a gene; a gene is expressed when its biological product is present and active.

142. **Gene frequency:** The frequency with which individuals in a population possess a particular gene; often confused with allele frequency.

143. **Gene Ontology Consortium:** Attempts to produce a dynamic controlled vocabulary that can be applied to all eukaryotes.

144. **Gene pool: Sum total of all** The different genes(alleles) in a population.

145. **Gene splicing:** The enzymatic attachment of one gene, or part of a gene, to another; also called splicing.

146. **Genetic code:** The complex process by which the information in RNA is decoded in to a polypeptide chain.

147. **Genetic counselling:** The process of identifying parents at risk, for producing children with genetic defects and of assessing the generic state of early embryos.

148. **Genetic engineering:** A technique for artificially and deliberately modifying DNA(genes) to suit human needs.

149. **Genetic Information:** The hereditary information contained in a sequence of nucleotide bases in chromosomal DNA or RNA.

150. **Genetic mapping:** A diagram showing the relative sequence and position of specific genes along a chromosome.

151. **Genetic Recombination:** Presence of a new combination of alleles in a DNA molecule compared to the parental genotype; the result of processes such as crossing over at meiosis, chromosome rearrangements, gene mutation and recombinant DNA technology.

152. **Genome:** Total number of genes contained in one haploid set of chromosomes of a diploid organism.

153. **Genome Database:** Regions of the human genome, including genes, clones, amplimers (PCR markers), breakpoints, cytogenetic markers, fragile sites, ESTs, syndromic regions, contigs and repeats. Maps of the human genome, including cytogenetic maps, linkage maps, radiation hybrid maps, content conting maps, and interested maps. These maps can be displayed

graphically via the web. Variations within the human genome including mutations and polymorphisms, plus allele frequency data.

154. **Genomic library:** DNA library consisting of fragments of chromosomal DNA.

155. **Genus, plural genera (Latin, for race):** A taxonomic category between family and species; includes one or more closely – related species; it form the first part of the binomial of the scientific name of organism and is written or printed with an initial capital letter.

156. **Geometric isomers:** Isomers related by rotation about a double bond; also called cis and trans isomers.

157. **Germ-**Line Cell: A type of animal cell that is formed early in embryogensesis and may multiply by mitosis or may produce, by meiosis, cell that develop into gametes (egg or sperm cells).

158. **Glycosylation:** The addition of sugar residues by modification of so,e protiens, that are released in the lumen and are incorporated in golgi vesicles.

159. **Gram molecular weight:** The weight in grams of a compound that is numerically equal to its molecular weight, the weight of one mole.

160. **Gram reaction:** A method of differential staining of bacteria by treating them with a special iodine solution after they have been stained with Gentian violet. Certain species of bacteria (gram-positive) retain the purple dye and others (gram-negative) are decolorized, thus affording a basis for classification.

161. **Growth Fork:** The region on a DNA duplex molecule where synthesis is taking place. It resembles a fork in shape, since it consists of a region of duplex DNA connected to a region of unwound single strands.

162. **Guanine:** A nitrogen base, one of the two pyrimidines found in DNA & RNA.

163. **Gyrase:** It is a type II topo isomerase of E.Coli with the ablility to introduce negative super coils in the DNA.

164. **Hairpin:** A double-helical stretch formed by base pairing between neighboring complementary sequences of a single strand of DNA or RNA.

165. **Half-life:** (1) For a chemical reaction, the time at which half of the substance has been consumed and turned into product. (2). In biochemistry, the time required for the disappearance or decay of one-half of a given component in a system. Half-lives vary from isotope to isotope, some being less than a millionth of a second and some more than a million years; symbol, $T_{1/2}$; also called half-time.

166. **Helicase:** The enzymes which help in unwinding of two strands of DNA.
167. **Helix:** Anything of a spiral shape; in biology, it refers to the shape of DNA molecules, which occur as double helices.
168. **Heredity:** The transmission of characters from one generation to successive generations of living things.
169. **Heterochromatin: (heteros^G = different + chroma^G = colour):** Region of a eukaryotic chromosome that remains permanently condensed and therefore is not transcribed into RNA; stains darkly with Giemsa stain; most centromere regions are heterochromatic; easily visible by light microscopy. Heterochromatin is either constitutive or facultative. Constitutive heterochromatin is composed of repeated sequences of DNA. Facultative heterochromatin is a transient form of inactive DNA (an inactive X chromosome, for example) that is usually the result of methylation of cytosine.
170. **Heteroduplex:** An annealed duplex structure between two DNA strands that do not show perfect complementarity. Can arise by mutation, recombination or the annealing of complementary single-stranded DNAs.
171. **Heterogeneous nuclear RNA (hn RNA):** The pool of primary RNA transcripts in the nucleus which are of various, usually large sizes. It is, in fact, the immediate product of transcription in an eukaryote, containing both introns and exons; also known as pre-mRNA.
172. **Heteropolymer:** A polymer that is made of more than one kind of monomer; for example, polypeptides and nucleic acids. Compare homopolymer.
173. **High-energy bond:** A covalent bond that has low activation energy and is broken easily and which on hydrolysis releases an unusually large amount of free energy under the conditions existing in a cell. A group linked to a molecule by such a bond is readily transferred from one molecule to another; common examples are the phosphodiester bonds in ATP and the thioester linkage in acetyl-CoA.
174. **Highly repetitive DNA:** It is the first component to reassociate and is equated with satellite DNA.
175. **Histone (histos^G = tissue):** The family of five very basic positively-charged, low-molecular-weight polypeptides, rich in arginine and lysine, that are tightly associated with DNA in the chromosomes of all eukaryotic cells. Histones form the core of nucleosomes, around which DNA is wrapped. The 5 major histones are represented as H1, H2A, H2B, H3, H4.
176. **Homeotic Genes:** Genes that regulate the development of the pattern of segment in the Droshphilia body plan; similar genes are found in most vertebrates.

177. **Homologous chromosome (homologia^G = agreement):** One of the two nearly identical versions of each chromosome. Chromosomes that associate in pairs in the first state of meiosis. In diploid cells, one chromosome of a pair that carry equivalent genes.

178. **Homologous Genetic Recombination:** Recombination between two DNA molecule of similar sequence. Occurring in all cells; occurs during meiosis and mitosis in eukaryotes.

179. **Homopolymer:** A polymer composed of only one type of monomeric building block.

180. **Homstrad:** A cured database of structure-based alignments for homologous protein families.

181. **Hotspot:** A site at which the frequency of mutation (or recombination) is very much increased.

182. **Human Transcript Database:** A curated source for information related to RNA molecule that have been sequenced.

183. **Housekeeping (constitutive) genes:** Gene that are expressed in all cells because they provide basic functions needed for sustenance of all cell types.

184. **Hybridization:** The specific reassociation of complementary strands of nuclei acids (DNA with DNA, DNA with RNA, or RNA with RNA).

185. **Hybridoma:** The pairing of complementary RNA and DNA strands to give an RNA-DNA hybrid.

186. **Hyperchromic Effect:** The large increase in light absorption at 260 nm occurring as a double-helical DNA is melted (unwound)

187. **Insert:** An additional length of base pairs in DNA, generally introduced by the techniques of recombinant DNA technology.

188. **Initiation Codon:** AUG (some times GUG in prokaryotes;) codes for the first amino acid in a polypeptide sequence: N-fromylmethionine in prokaryotes, and methionine in eukaryotes.

189. **Initiation Factors:** Those protein factors that are speciafically required during the initiation phase of protein synthesis.

190. **Intercalating Agent:** A chemical, usually containing aromatic rings, that can sandwich in between adjacent base pairs in a DNA duplex. The intercalation leads to an adjustment in the DNA secondary structure, as adjacent base pairs ar usually close-packed.

191. **Intercalating Mutagen:** A mutagen that inserts itself between two successive bases in a nucleic acid, causing a frame shift mutation.

192. **Intron:** Those regions of a gene which do not have the information for a protien.

193. **Inversion:** They are and additional stretch of base pairs in DNA.

194. **Inverted terminal repeats:** These are the short related or identical sequence present in reverse orientation at the ends of some transposon.

195. **In vitro (Latin, for "in glass"):** A term used by biochemists to describe a process taking place in an isolated cell-free extract. Also used by cell biologists to refer to cells growing in culture usually taken in glass equipments as opposed to in an organism (in vivo).

196. **In vivo *Latin, for "in life"):** Refers to a process taking place in an intact (i.e., living) cell or an organism, as opposed to in a culture (in vitro).

197. **Initiation complex:** A complex of a ribosome with an mRNA and the initiating Met-tRNA ^{Met} or fMet-tRNA ^{fMet}, the formation of which begins polypeptide (or protein) synthesis.

198. **Initiation codon:** AUG (sometimes GUG in prokaryotes); codes for the first amino acid in a polypeptide sequence; N-formylmethionine in prokaryotes and methionine in eukaryotes; also called start codon.

199. **Initiation factor:** A protein that promotes the proper association of ribosomes with mRNA and is required for the initiation of protein synthesis.

200. **Intron: (intra^L = within):** A noncoding sequence of nucleotides within a eukaryotic gene that is transcribed into an mRNA molecule but is then excised by RNA splicing before the gene is translated. These untranslated regions of DNA make up the bulk of most eukaryotic genes; also called as intervening sequence. Compare exon.

201. **Karyotype (karyon^G = kernel + typos^G = stamp or print):** Full set of chromosomes of a cell arranged with respect to size, shape and number.

202. **Kilobase(Kb):** It is an abbreviation for 1000 base pairs of DNA or 1000 base pairs of RNA.

203. **KEGG (Kyoto Encyclopedia of Genes and Genomes):** Information pathways that consist of interacting molecule or genes and to provide links from the gene catalogs produced by genome sequencing projects.

204. **Kinase:** An enzyme that catalyzes the transfer of a high energy group from a donar usually ATP to an acceptor and named according to the acceptor as creatine kinase, fructokinase, etc An enzyme that activates a zymogen and named according to its source as enterokinase, streptokinase, etc.

205. **Lac operon:** A cluster of genes encoding 3 proteins that bacteria use to obtain energy from the sugar lactose.

206. **Lagging strand:** One of the two newly-made strands of DNA found at a replication fork. The lagging strand is synthesized in the direction opposite

to that in which the replication fork moves and is made in discontinuous lengths that are later joined covalently. Compare leading strand.

207. **Lambrush chromosome:** Gaint diplotene chromosome found in the oocyte nucleus. The loops that are observed are the sites of extensive gene expression.

208. **Leader sequence:** (1) For an mRNA, the nontranslated sequence at the 5' ends of the molecule that precedes the initiation codon. (2) For a protein, a short, hydrophobic sequence of amino acids from amino terminal that signals the cellular fate or destination of a newly-synthesized protein, also called signal sequence.

209. **Leader strand:** One of the two newly-made strands of DNA found at a replication fork. The leading strand is synthesized in the same direction in which the replication fork moves and is made by continuous synthesis in the 5' → 3' direction. Compare lagging strand.

210. **Library:** A collection of cloned fragments that represents, in aggregate, the entire genome. Libraries may be either genomic DNA (in which both introns and exons are represented) or cDNA (in which only exons are represented).

211. **Ligation:** The enzyme-catalyzed joining in phosphodiester linkage of two stretches of DNA or RNA into one; the respective enzymes are DNA and RNA ligases.

212. **Ligase:** An enzyme that joins together (ligates) two molecules in an energy-dependent process. DNA ligase, for example, links two DNA molecules together through a phosphodiester bond.

213. **Ligation:** The joining of 2 DNA molecules with a covalent bond.

214. **Lines:** Long interspersed repeat sequences.

215. **Liposomes:** Concentric spheres of phospholipid bilayers.

216. **Luxury genes:** Genes coding for specialized functions synthesized (usually) in large amounts in particular cell types.

217. **Lysogeny:** One of two outcomes of the infection of a host cell by a temperature phage. It occurs when the phage genome becomes repressed and is replicated as part of the host DNA; infrequently it may be induced, and the phage particle so produced cause the host cell to lyse.

218. **M Phase:** That period of the cell cycle when mitosis takes place.

219. **Marker:** Any gene of interest in an experiment. Material inheritance describes the preferential survival in the progency of a cross of gentic markers provided by one parent.

220. **Melting Temperature**:(tm) is the midpoint of the temperature range over which DNA is denatured.

221. **Messenger RNA (mRNA):** A class of RNA molecules, each of which is complementary to one strand of DNA and which passes from the nucleus to the cytoplasm carries the genetic message of genes from the chromosomes to the ribosome's in the cytoplasm, where the message is translated into the amino acid sequence of a polypeptide.

222. **Microsatellite polymorphism:** Heterozygosis of a certain microsatellite repeat in an individual.

223. **Microsatellite repeat sequences:** Dispersed or group repeat sequences of 2-5 bp repeated up to 50 times. May occur at 50 – 100 thousands locations in the genome.

224. **Micron:** A unit of measurement: 1/1000 mm usually designated by the Greek letter μ.

225. **miRNAs:** MicroRNAs, 21 – 22 nucleotide long RNA species derived from RNA polymerase II transcription units, 500 – 1500 bp in length via RNA processing. These RNAs, recently discovered, are thought to play crucial roles in gene regulation.

226. **Mismatch Repair:** The replacement of a base in a heteroduplex structure by one that forms a Watson-Crick base pair.

227. **Missense Mutation:** A change in which a codon for one amino acid is replaced by codon for another amino acid.

228. **Mobile Genetic Element:** A segment of the genome that can move as a unit from one location on the genome to another, without any requirement for sequence homology.

229. **Molecular genetics:** Field of genetics devoted to the study of teh biochemical mechanisms by which heredity information is stored in nucleic acid and transmitted to proteins.

230. **Molecular weight (Mol.wt. or MW):** Numerically, the same as the relative molecular mass of a molecule, expressed in daltons alternatively, the sum of the atomic weight of the atoms in a molecule.

231. **Mutagen (mutare^L = to change):** A chemical or some other agent that causes mutations.

232. **Mutagenesis:** A process that leads to a change in the genetic material that is inherited in later generations.

233. **Mutant (mutare^L = to change):** A mutated gene. An organism carrying a gene that has undergone a mutation.

234. **Mutation (mutare^L = to change):** A permanent heritable changes in the DNA molecule of an organism.

235. **NDP(Nucleic Acid Database Project):** It assembles and distributes structural information about nucleic acids.

236. **Nascent RNA:** The initial transcripts of RNA, before any modification or processing.

237. **Nick:** A single-stranded cut or break in a DNA molecule; nicking of DNA may form part of a DNA repair mechanism, as occurs after damage caused by ultraviolet light.

238. **Nick translation:** A technique for labeling DNA based on the ability of DNA polymerase from E coli to degrade a strand of DNA that has been nicked and then to resynthesize the strand: if a radioactive nucleoside triphosphate is employed, the rebuilt strand becomes labeled and can be used as a radioactive probe.

239. **Negative Supercoiling:** It refers to the twisting of a duplex of DNA in space in the opposite sense to the turns of the strands in the double helix.

240. **Northern blot:** A method for transferring RNA from an agarose or polyacrylamide gel to a nitrocellulose filter, on which the RNA can be detected by a suitable probe.

241. **Nonsense codon:** It is the any one of the 3 triplets (UAG,UAA and UGA) that cause termination of protein synthesis.

242. **Nonsense Mutation:** A change in the base sequence that converts a sense codon (one that specifies an amino acid) to one that specifies a stop (a nonsense codon).

243. **Non sense Suppressor:** A mutation, usually in the gene for a tRNA, that causes an aminoacid to be inserted into a polypeptide in response to a termination codon.

244. **Nucleoplasm:** The portion of cells contents enclosed b y the nuclear membrane; also called as nuclear matrix.

245. **Nucleoside:** A compound composed of a purine or pyrimidine base covalently linked to a pentose sugar, either a ribose (ribonucleoside) or a deoxyribose (deoxyribonucleoside).

246. **Nucleases:** Enzyme that depolymerize nucleic acids.

247. **Nucleosome (nucleus^L = kernel + soma^L = body):** The structural, packaging unit of a eukaryotic chromosome, composed of a short DNA strand wrapped around a core of histone proteins; the fundamental subunit of chromatin.

248. **Nucleoid:** In bacteria, the nuclear zone that contains the chromosome but has no surrounding membrane.

249. **Nuclear sap:** The fluid which is lost by the chromosomes as they contact during prophase and which fills the space of nucleus

250. **Nucleotide:** A monomeric unit of nucleic acids, composed of a phosphate, a pentose sugar (ribose or deoxyribose) and a nitrogenous base (purine or pyrimidine); DNA and RNA are polymers of nucleotides. Alternatively, a nucleotide is a nucleoside with one or more phosphate groups joined in ester linkages to the sugar moiety.

251. **Nucleolus:** A body in the nucleus which disappear and does not resolve itself into chromosomes at mitosis.

252. **Nucleus, plural nuclei (Latin, for a kernel, dim. Fr. Nux = nut):** In a eukaryotic cell, a promenent, membrane-bounded organelle that contains chromosomes; the nucleus is the repository of the genetic information that directs all activities of a living cell. In atoms, the central core, containing positively-charged protons and (in all but hydrogen) electrically-neutral neutrons.

253. **Nucleophile:** An electron rich group with a strong tendency to donate electrons to an electrons –deficient nucleus (electrophile); the entering reactant in a biomolecular substitution reaction

254. **Nucleic acids:** DNA+RNA found in the nucleus. These are compounds of a molecule of phosphoric acid, sugar and a nitrogenous base (either a purine or a pyrimidine)

255. **Ochre Codon:** The triplet UAA, one of three nonsense codons that cause termination of protein synthesis.

256. **Okazaki fragments (after R. Okazaki, the discoverer):** Newly synthesized Short fragments of DNA that are formed on the lagging strand of DNA during replication.

257. **Oligonucleotide:** A short, defined sequence of nucleotides joined together in the typical phosphodiester linkage.

258. **Oncogene theory (oncos^G = tumour):** The hypothesis that cancer results from the action of a specific tumor-inducing onc gene.

259. **One-gene/one-enzyme hypothesis:** The hypothesis that genes produce their effects by specifying the structure of enzymes and that each gene encodes the structure of a enzymes and that each gene encodes the structure of a single enzyme; put forward by George Beadle and Edward Tatum in 1941.

260. **Ontogeny:** The whole of the development of an organism from fertilization to the completion of life history.

261. **Open reading frame (ORF):** A group of contiguous nonoverlapping nucleotide codons in a DNA or RNA molecule between an initiation codon and a termination codon. It represents the coding sequence for a polypeptide.

262. **Operator:** Gene that regulates the activity of structural genes.

263. **Operon (operis^L = work):** The structural genes and an operator made an operon.

264. **Ori:** The origin of DNA replication.

265. **PAC:** A high-capacity (70 – 95 kb) cloning vector based upon the lytic E coli bacteriophage P1 that replicates in bacteria as an extrachromosomal element.

266. **Palindrome:** A sequence of duplex DNA that is the same when the two strands are read in opposite directions. For example TGAC in the following DNA segment:
    i.   5' XXX TGAC XXX 3'
    ii. 3' XXX CAGT XXX 5'

267. **Pentose:** A simple sugar with a backbone containing five carbon atoms.

268. **Phenotype: the visible expression of the hereditary constitution possessed by an organism.**

269. **Plasmid:** A small. Extrachromosomal, circular molecule of DNA that replicates independently of the host DNA.

270. **PMD (Protein Mutant Database):** It covers natural as well as artificial mutants, including random and site-directed ones, for all protein except members of the globin and immunoglobulin familes.

271. **Poly-A tail:** A chain of adenylic acid molecules that is added to a molecule of RNA immediately after it has been transcribed and cleaved from its DNA template.

272. **Polymerase:** An enzyme that catalyzes the joining of DNA or RNA nucleotides.

273. **Polymerase chain reaction (PCR):** An enzymatic method for the repeated copying (and thus amplification) of the two strands of DNA that make up a particular gene sequence.

274. **Polymerization: (polus^G = many + meris^G = part + izein^G = to combine with):** A process in which many small identical subunits (monomers) combine to one another chemically to form a long chain of a polymer molecule.

275. **Polymorphism (polys^G = many + meris^G form):** The presence of distinctly different, genetically-determined phenotypic characteristics within a population of a single species.

276. **Polynucleotide:** A covalently-linked sequence of nucleotides in which the 3' hydroxyl of the pentose of one nucleotide residue is joined by a phosphodiester bond to the 5' hydroxyl of the pentose of the next residue.

277. **Polysome or(polyribosome):** The series of ribosomes translating the same single strand of mRNA.

278. **Polytene Chromosomes:** A giant chromosome fromed by successive replication of a chromosome set without separation of the replicas.

279. **Positive supercoiling:** It refers to the coiling of the double helix in space in the same n direction as the winding of the two stands of the double helix itself.

280. **Positive regulator proteins:** Proteins required for the activation of a transcription unit.

281. **Posttranslational modification:** Enzyme-catalyzed changes (or) modifications in a polypeptide chain after it is synthesized (or translated) from its mRNA; the various modifications include cleavage, glycosylation, phosphorylation, methylation, and prenylation.

282. **Posttranscriptional processing:** The enzymatic processing of the primary RNA transcript, producing functional mRNA, tRNA and/or rRNA molecules.

283. **Print:** (Protein Fingerprint Database) a compendium of protein fingerprints. A fingerprint is a group of conserved motifs used to characterize a protein family.

284. **Primary transcript:** The immediate RNA product of transcription before any post transcriptional processing reactions.

285. **Primase:** It polymerises ribonucleotide bases in the formation of a primer.

286. **Primer:** This is a short RNA segment formed on DNA template prior to the beginning of replication.

287. **Primosome:** The mobile complex of helicase and primase that is involved in DNA replication.

288. **Prinow box:** The consensus sequence TATAAATG centered about 10bp before the startpoint of bacterial genes. It is a part of the promoter especially important in binding RNA polymerase.

289. **Probe:** DNA strands with specific nucleotide sequences complementary to VNTR (Variable Number Tandem Repeats) sequences.

290. **Prokaryote (pro^G = before + karyon^G = kernel):** A unicellular organism with a single chromosome, no nuclear envelope, no membrane-bounded organelles and no mitosis or meiosis; prokaryotes include bacteria and cyan bacteria; also spelt as procaryote; compare eukaryote.

291. **Promoter:** Gene that forms the binding site of RNA polymerase.

292. **Proofreading:** The ability of DNA polymerases to remove mismatched nucleotides with 3' to 5' exonuclease activity during DNA synthesis.

293. **Prophase:** A phase genome covalently integrated as a linear part of the bacterial chromosome.

294. **Proteome:** The entire collection of expressed proteins in an organism.

295. **Pseudogene:** An inactive segment of DNA arising by mutation of a parental active gene; typically generated by transposition of a cDNA copy of an mRNA.

296. **Psoriasis:** (from a Greek word, meaning to have the itch): A noncontagious disease of the skin marked by scaly red patches, due probably to a disorder of the immune system.

297. **Pyranose:** A simple sugar containing 6-membered pyrane ring.

298. **Purine:** Double-ring, nitrogen –containing base which is an important component of DNA and RNA and certain other biologically active substances. Two purines, the adenine and guanine, are found in both DNA and RNA.

299. **Pyrimidine:** A nitrogenous heterocyclic base serving as a component of nucleotide or nucleic acid.

300. **Pyrimidine dimer:** A covalently-joined dimer of two adjacent pyrimidine residues in DNA, induced by absorption of ultraviolet light; most commonly derived from two adjacent thymine's (a thymine dimer).

301. **Pyrophosphate:** An enzyme hydrolyzing inorganic pyrophosphophate to yield 2 molecules of phosphate (orthophosphate).

302. **Pyrophosphate Cleavage:** Enzymatic cleavage of ATP to yield AMP and pyrophosphate.

303. **Radiation:** The electromagnetic energy that travels through empty space with the speed of the light (2×10^8 ms^{-1}). All objects emit radiation, at room temperature mostly in the infrared range. Whereas at high temperatures visible radiation is produced.

304. **Rebonucleotide:** A nucleotide containing D-ribose as its pentose component.

305. **Recombinant DNA:** - DNA produced by joining together genes from different sources.

306. **Recombination:** A process in which chromosomes or DNA molecules are broken and the fragments are rejoined in new combinations. In bacteria, it is accomplished by the transfer of genes into cells, often in association with viruses. In eukaryotes, it is accomplished by reassortment of chromosomes during meiosis and by crossing-over.

307. **Recombinantion repair:** It is a mode of filling a gap in one strand of the duplex DNA by retrieving a homologous single strand from another duplex.

308. **Ribonucleic acid:** A kind of nucleic acid found mainly in the cytoplasm but a little in the nucleus. It brings about the synthesis of protein and helps in translating the genetic information of DNA in t action.

309. **Regulatory gene:** A gene that codes for an RNA or protein product whose function is to control the expression of other genes.

310. **Renaturation:** It is the association of denatured complementary single strand of DNA double helix.

311. **Repetition frequency:** The number of copies of a given sequence present in the haploid genome.

312. **Replication:** Y-shaped region of a replicating DNA molecule at which the two daughter strands are formed and separate.

313. **Replication origin:** The point of initiation of DNA synthesis along the double helix; two replication forks form at the replication origin and move in opposite directions from one another during DNA synthesis.

314. **Replication fork:** The point at which strands of parentral duplex DNA are separated so that replication can proceed.

315. **Replicon:** A black of DNA capable of replication (for example, a plasmid or a chromosome).

316. **Replisome:** The multiprotein complex that promotes DNA synthesis at the replication fork.

317. **Repetitive DNA:** Sequences of DNA that occur in many copies in a genome; some sequences of repetitive DNA can occur in a million copies per nucleus.

318. **Repression:** The ability of bacteria to prevent synthesis of certain enzymes when their products are present; more generally, refers to inhibition of transcription (or translation) by binding of repressor protein to specific site on DNA (or mRNA).

319. **Restriction endonuclease:** Any such enzyme which very specifically recognises a perticular DNA sequence, and cuts it. These enzymes are the molecular scissors.

320. **Restriction enzyme:** An endodeoxynuclease that causes cleavage of both strands of DNA at highly specific sites dictated by the base sequence.

321. **Restriction fragment:** A segment of double-stranded DNA produced by the action of a restriction endonuclease on a larger DNA.

322. **Restriction map:** Diagrammatic representation of a DNA molecule indicating the sites of cleavage by various restriction endonucleases.

323. **Retrovirus (retro^L = turning back):** An RNA virus containing a reverse transcriptase and that which replicates in a cell by first making a double-stranded DNA intermediate, which it can then insert into the cellular DNA as if it were a cellular gene. Human immunodeficiency virus (HIV) is a common example.

324. **Reverse transcription:** RNA-directed synthesis of DNA, catalyzed by reverse transcriptase.

325. **Rho factor:** A protein involved in assisting E.Coli RNA polymerase to terminate transcription at certain (rho-dependent) sites.

326. **Ribonuclease:** A nuclease that catalyzes the hydrolysis of certain internucleotide linkages of RNA.

327. **Ribonucleic acid, RNA:** A polynucleotide having a specific sequence of ribonucleotide units covalently joined through 3', 5' – phosphodiester bonds; molecules of RNA, which are made as complements of DNA segments called genes, function in protein synthesis; differentiated into 3 types: mRNA, rRNA and tRNA.

328. **Ribose:** A 5-carbon sugar with one oxygen atom more than the related sugar deoxyribose; a component of ribonucleic acid.

329. **Ribosomal RNA (rRNA):** A class of RNA molecules serving as components of ribosomes and often distinguished by their sedimentation coefficient, such as 28 s rRNA or 5 s rRNA; participate in the synthesis of proteins.

330. **Ribosome:** A cell organelle composed of rRNAs and proteins (approximately 18 to 22 mm in diameter) that are arranged in two subunits, one large and one small; prokaryotes have ribosomes with 70 s size and mass and eukaryotes have large ribosomes with 80 s size and mass; ribosome associates with mRNA and catalyzes the synthesis of proteins.

331. **Ribozymes:** Ribonucleic acid molecules with catalytic activities; RNA enzymes.

332. **Ribulose ($C_5H_{10}O_5$):** A ketopentose sugar, found in syrup; plays important role in carbohydrate metabolism.

333. **RNA polymerase:** An enzyme that catalyze the synthesis of an RNA molecule from ribonucleoside 5'-triphosphate precursors, using a strand of DNA or RNA as a template.

334. **RNA Cribonucleic acid:** Single-stranded polynucleotide chain having ribose sugar.

335. **RT-PCR:** A method used to quantitative mRNA levels that relies upon a first step of cDNA copying of mRNAs catalyzed by reverse transcriptase prior to PCR amplification and quantitation.

336. **Salvage pathway:** Synthesis of a biomolecule (such as a nucleotide) from intermediates in the degradative pathway for the biomolecule; a recycling pathway, as distinct from a de novo pathway.

337. **Satellite DNA:** DNA consisting of multiple tandem repeats of very short, simple nucleotide sequences; makes up to 10 to 20% of genome of higher eukaryotes; usually identifiable by its unusual nucleotide composition; most often associated with the centromeric region; satellite DNA is not transcribed and has no known function.

338. **Semiconservative replication:** It is accomplished by the separation of the strands of parentral duplex, each other acting as a template for the synthesis of a complementary strand.

339. **Sex-chromosomes:** Chromosomes which exhibit difference either in shape or in number in male and female sexes, or which are concerned with the determination of sex,e.g. X and Y chromosomes.

340. **Shine-Dalgarno sequence:** It consists of many tandem (identical or related) of a short basic repeating unit.

341. **Shotgun experiment:** Cloning of an entire genome in the form of randomly generated fragments.

342. **Signal:** The end product observed when a specific sequence of DNA or RNA is detected by autoradiography or some other method. Hybridization with a complementary radioactive polynucleotide (eg, by Southern or Northern blotting) is commonly used to generate th e signal.

343. **Sigma factor:** The subunit of bacterial RNA polymerase needed for initiation; is the major influence on selection of binding sites (promoters).

344. **Sines:** Short interspersed repeat sequences.

345. **SiRNAs:** Silencing RNAs, 21 – 25 nt in length generated by selective nucleolytic degradation of double – stranded RNAs of cellular or viral origin. SiRNAs anneal to various specific sites within target in RNAs leading to mRNA degradation, hence gene "knockdown."

346. **SNP:** Single nucleotide polymorphism. Refers to the fact that single nucleotide genetic variation in genome sequence exists at discrete loci throughout the chromosomes. Measurement of allelic SNP differences is useful for gene mapping studies.

347. **snRNA:** Small nuclear RNA. This family of RNAs is best known for its role in mRNA processing.

348. **Somatic cell (soma^G = body):** Any cell of a plant or animal other than a germ cell or germ-cell precursor.

349. **Southern blot:** A method for transferring DNA from an agarose gel to nitrocellulose filter, on which the DNA can be detected by a suitable probe to a transfer membrane that contains a renatured protein.

350. **Spliceosome:** The macromolecular complex responsible for precursor mRNA splicing. The spliceosome consists of at least five small nuclear RNAs (snRNA; U1, U2, U4, U5, and U6) and many proteins.

351. **Splicing:** The removal of introns from RNA accompanied by the joining of its exons.

352. **Staggered cuts:** Cuts in duplex DNA are made when two strands are cleaved at different points near each other producing sticky ends.

353. **Sticky-jended DNA:** Complementary single strands of DNA that protrude from opposite ends of a DNA duplex or from the ends of difference duplex molecules (see also Blunt – ended DNA, above).

354. **Stop codons:** RNA codons that signal a ribosome a strop tranlating an mRNA and to release the polypeptide. In the normal genetic code, there are 3 stop codon,: UAA, UAG and UGA.

355. **Stringent replication:** The limitation of single –copy plasmids replication pari passu with the bacterial chromosomes.

356. **Structural gene:** A gene or a regions of DNA that codes for a protein or RNA molecule and consequently the protein, as distinct from a regulatory gene that regulates gene expression.

357. **Supercoiled DNA:** A region of DNA in which the double helix is further twisted on itself.

358. **Syndrome:** A group of symptoms appearing together for a perticular condition.

359. **Synergism:** A chemical phenomenon in which the combined activity of two or more compounds is greater than the sum of the individual activities. For example, auxin and cytokinin act synergistically in promoting DNA replication.

360. **Tandem:** Used to describe multiple copies of the same sequence (eg, DNA) that lie adjacent to one another.

361. **Target cell:** Any cell that responds to specific hormones.

362. **TATA box:** Consensus sequence in the promoter region of many eukaryotic genes that binds a general transcription factor and hence specifies the position where transcription is initiated.

363. **Temperature:** The degrees of hotness of coldness, usually related to a zero at teh melting point or ice (Celsius scale) or absolute zero (Kelvin scale).

364. **Template:** A macromolecular mould or pattern for the syn thesis of an informational macromolecule.

365. **Tendon (tenon^G = stretch):** A bunch of parallel collagen fibers making up a band of connective tissue which serves to attach a muscle to a bone.

366. **Terminal transferase:** An enzyme that adds nucleotides of one type (eg, deoxyadenonucleotidyl residues) to the 3' end of DNA strands.

367. **Termination codons:** UAA, UAG and UGA; in protein synthesis, these three codon signal the termination of a polypeptide chain; also known as stop codon s or nonsense codons.

368. **Termination factors:** Protein factors of the cytosol required in releasing a completed polypeptide chain from a ribosome; also known as release factors.

369. **Termination sequence:** A DNA sequence that appears at the end of a transcriptional unit and signals the end of transcription.

370. **Thymine:** A pyrimidine occuring in DNA but not in RNA; always base-pairs with a DNA purine base called adenine.

371. **Transcript:** A RNA product of DNA transcription.

372. **Transduction:** (1) Generally, the conversion of energy or information from one forms to another 2) The transfer of DNA from one bacterium to another, using a virus as a vector.

373. **Transcription:** Template DNA directed synthesis of nucleic acids; typically DNA-directed synthesis of RNA.

374. **Transcriptome:** The entire collection of expressed mRNAs in an organism.

375. **Transfection:** Introduction of a foreign DNA molecule into a eukaryotic cell; usually followed into a eukaryotic cell; usually followed by expression of one or more genes in the newly-introduced DNA.

376. **Transfer RNA, tRNA (trans^L = across + ferre^L = to bear or carry):** A class of small molecules (M.W.25,000 – 30,000) that float free in the cytoplasm and each of which combines covalently with a specific amino acid and to

a codon on messenger RNA and later transfers the amino acid to mRNA in ribosome for assembly into proteins.

377. **Transferase:** Any enzyme that catalyzes the transfer of a chemical group (such as amino, methyl or alkyl) from one substrate to another substrate.

378. **Transformation (trans^L = across + formare^L = to shape):** (1) The incorporation of a piece of foreign DNA into the genome of a bacterial cell, causing the recipient to acquire a new phenotype. The process is important historically since, following transformation experiments by Frederick Griffith on Pneumococcus bacterium, DNA was shown to be the genetic material of cell by Avery, MacLeod and McCarthy. (2) In the case of cultured animal cells, the term usually refers to the acquisition of cancer like properties following treatment with a virus or a carcinogen.

379. **Transgenic:** genetically modified organism (GMO) carrying foreign genes. The introduced foreign gene is called transgene.

380. **Translation (trans^L = across + latus^L = that which is carried):** The process by which the sequence of nucleotides in a messenger RNA molecule directs the incorporation of amino acids into protein; occurs on a ribosome. Compare transcription.

381. **Translational repressor:** A repressor that binds to an mRNA, blocking translation.

382. **Transgenic:** Genetically modified organisms (GMO) carrying foreign genes. The introduced foreign gene is called transgene.

383. **Translation:** Synthesis of protein using mRNA as template.

384. **Uracil:** A nitrogen base of RNA.

385. **Uric acid, $C_5H_4O_3N_4$:** An organic compound belonging to the purine group; a colourless crystalline solid that is slightly soluble in water; occurs in very small amounts in the urine of some animals (reptiles) as a breakdown product of amino acids and nucleic acids; being quite insoluble in water, it is thus nontoxic when released during embryonic development within the egg; also permits the removal of nitrogen with a minimum of water loss and is eliminated as a thick paster or even dry pellets; sodium and potassium salts of the acid are deposited in the joints in cases of gout.

386. **Vector:** An intermidiate carrier (in genetic engineering), a phage, plasmid or virus DNA in to which another DNA is inserted for introduction in to bacterial or other cells for amplification (DNA cloning).

387. **Virus:** An ultramicroscopic pathogenic particle, capable of passing through bacteriological filters; consists of nucleic acid (DNA or RNA) enclosed in a protein coat; capable of replicating within a living host cells only and

spreading from cell to cell; infect cells of bacteria, plants and animals, and whilst viruses carry out no metabolism themselves, they are able to control the metabolism of the infected cell.

388. **Western blot:** A method for transferring protein to a nitrocellulose filter, on which the protein can be detected by a suitable probe (eg, an antibody).

389. **3' end:** The end of a nucleic acid that lacks a nucleotide bound at the 3' position of the terminal residue.

390. **5' end:** The end of a nucleic acid that lacks a nucleotide bound at the 5' position of the terminal residue.

Appendix 1

S.NO:	Greek letter	Greek name	Greek equivalent
1)	A, α	Alpha	a
2)	B, β	Beta	b
3)	Γ,γ	Gamma	g
4)	Δ,δ	Delta	d
5)	E, ε	Epsilon	ĕ
6)	Z, ζ	Zeta	z
7)	H, η	Eta	ē
8)	Θ,θ	Theta	th
9)	I, ι	Iota	i
10)	K, κ	Kappa	k
11)	Λ,λ	Lambda	I
12)	M, μ	Mu	m
13)	N, ν	Nu	n
14)	Ξ, ξ	Xi	x
15)	O,o	Omricron	o
16)	Π,π	Pi	p
17)	P,ρ	Rho	r
18)	Σ,σ	Sigma	s
19)	T,τ	Tau	t
20)	Y,υ	Upsilon	u
21)	Φ,φ	Phi	ph
22)	X,χ	Chi	ch
23)	Ψ,ψ	Psi	Ps
24)	Ω,ω	Omega	ō

Greek letter	Greek name	Greek equivalent
A, α	Alpha	a
B, β	Beta	b
Γ,γ	Gamma	g
Δ,δ	Delta	d
E, ε	Epsilon	ĕ
Z, ζ	Zeta	z
H, η	Eta	ē
Θ,θ	Theta	th
I, ι	Iota	i
K, κ	Kappa	k
Λ,λ	Lambda	I
M, μ	Mu	m
N, ν	Nu	n
Ξ, ξ	Xi	x
O,o	Omricron	o
Π,π	Pi	p
P,ρ	Rho	r
Σ,σ	Sigma	s
T,τ	Tau	t
Y,υ	Upsilon	u
Φ,φ	Phi	ph
X,χ	Chi	ch
Ψ,ψ	Psi	Ps
Ω,ω	Omega	ō

The 8 Base Units

1. Length	Metre	m
2. Mass	Kilogram	kg
3. Time	Second	s
4. Amount of substance	Mole	mol

5. Thermodynamic temperature Kelvin   K

6. Electric current   Ampere   A

7. Luminous intensity   Candela   cd

8. Katalytic amount   Katal   kat

COMPARISON OF METRIC AND OTHER UNITS

1 centimetre	= 0.3937 inch	1 inch	= 2.5400 centimetres
1 mitre	= 3.2808 feet	1 foot	= 0.30480 metre
1 metre	= 1.09367 yards	1 yard	= 0.91440 metre
1 kilometre	= 0.62137 mile	1 mile	= 1.60934 kilometres

Units of Area

1 square cm	= 0.1550 sq. In.	1 square in.	= 6.4516 sq.cm.
1 square metre	= 10.7638 sq.ft.	1 square ft.	= 0.9290 sq.m.
1 square metre	= 1.1960 sq.yds.	1 square yd.	= 0.83613 sq.m.
1 square km.	= 0.38610 sq. mile	1 square mile	= 2.5900 sq. km.
1 hectare	= 2.47105 acres	1 acre	= 0.40469 hectare

Units of Volume

1 cubic cm. (c.c.)	= 0.061024 cubic in.	1 cubic in.	= 16.387 c.c.
1 cubic m.	= 35.3144 cubic ft.	1 cubic ft.	= 0.028317 cubic m.
1 cubic m.	= 1.3079 cubic yds.	1 cubic yd.	= 0.7645 cubic m.

Measures of Liquid Capacity

British Units (or Imperial Units)

Penny weight	= 3.858 carats
1 gallon	= 4 quarts = 8 pints = 32 gills
1 gallon	= 4.54596 litres
1 litre	= 0.2200 gallon = 1.7598 pints

U.S. Units

1 gallon	= 4 quarts = 8 pints = 32 gills
1 gallon	= 3.78533 litres

Apothecaries' Units (British)

1 gallon	= 8 pints = 160 fluid ounces
1 fluid ounce	= 8 fluid drachms = 24 scruples = 480 minims
1 gallon	= 4.54596 litres
1 litre	= 0.2200 gallon = 35.196 fluid ounces

Apothecaries' Units (U.S.)

1 gallon	= 8 pints	= 128 fluid ounces
1 fluid ounce	= 8 fluid drachms = 480 minims	
1 gallon	= 3.78533 litres	
1 litre	= 0.26418 gallon = 33.81504 fluid ounces	

Units of Mass

Avoiduposis Weight. This is a British and American system of weights, based on a pound of 16 ounces.

1 hundredweight	= 4 squarters = 8 stones = 112 pounds
1 pound	= 16 ouncfes = 256 drachms = 7,000 grains
1 grain	= 0.064799 g
1 grain	= 15.4323 grains
1 hundredweight	= 50.80238 kg
1 kilogram	= 0.0198461 hundredweight
1 millier	= 1 metric ton = 10 quintals
1 quintal	= 10 myriagram = 100 kilogram = 0.09842059 ton
1 kilogram	= 2.204621 pounds
1 pounds	= 0.4535926 kilogram

Troy Weight. This is a system of weights, used for gems and precious metals (gold, silver) and also for drugs.

1 pound	= 12 ounces = 240 pennyweights

1 pennyweight (dwt.)	= 6 carats = 24 grains
1 gram	= 0.3215 ounce = 0.643
Pennyweight = 3.858 carats	
1 carats	= 0.25920 gram

Apothecaries's Weight - This is a system of weights, used in pharmacy.

1 pound	= 12 ounces = 96 drachms
1 drachm	= 3 scruples = 60 grains
1 gram	= 0.03215 ounce = 0.2572
Drachm = 0.7716 scruple	
1 scruple	= 1.29598 gram

Mathematical Signs and Symbols

=	equals
≈Ξ	equals approximately
≠	is not equal to
Ξ	is identical to, is defined as
>	is greater than
»	is much greater than
<	is less than
≥	is more than or equal to
≤	is less than or equal to
±	plus or minus (e.g., $\sqrt{4} = +2$)
∞	is proportional to
Σ	the sum of

NUCLEIC ACIDS AND RELATED COMPOUNDS

A. Nitrogenous bases

A, Ade	Adenine
B	5-bromouracil
C,Cyt	Cytosine
G,Gua	Guanine
MC	Methylcytosine
T,Thy	Thymine
U,Ura	Uracil

B. Nitrogenous base derivatives

DiHu	5, 6-dihydrouracil
DiMeA	6-dimethyladenine
2-DiMeG	2-dimethylguanine
HMC	5-hydroxymethylcytosine
6-IPA	6-N-isopentenyladenine
6-MeA	6-methyladenine
5-MeC	5-methylcytosine

C. Nucleosides

Ribonucleosides

AR, Ado	Adenine ribonucleoside	Adenosine
CR, Cyd	Cytosine ribonucleoside	Cytidine
GR, Guo	Guanine ribonucleoside	Guanosine
TR, Thd	Thymine ribonucleoside	Thymidine
UR, Urd	Uracil ribonucleoside	Uridine

Deosyribonucleosides

AdR	Adenine deosyribonucleoside	Deoxyadenosine
CdR	Cytosine deoxyribonucleoside	Deoxycytidine
GdR	Guanine deoxyribonucleoside	Deoxyguanosine
TdR	Thymine deoxyribonucleoside	Deoxythymidine
UdR	Uracil deoxyribonucleoside	Deoxyuridine

D. Nucleoside phosphates (=nucleotides)

Adenosine	A, Ado	AMP	ADP	ATP
Cytidine	C, Cyd	CMP	CDP	CTP
Guanosine	G,Guo	GMP	GDP	GTP
Inosine	I, Ino	IMP	IDP	ITP
Thymidine	T, Thd	TMP	TDP	TTP
Uridine	U, Urd	UMP	UDP	UTP

E. Related compounds

DHU, UH_2	Dihydrouridine
DNA	Deoxyribonucleic acid
cDNA	Complementary DNA

mDNA	Inosine
mtDNA	Mitochondrial DNA
RNA	Ribonucleic acid
hnRNA	Heterogeneous nuclear RNA
mRNA	Messenger RNA or template RNA
nRNA	Ribosomal RNA
ns	Nucleoside (s)
nt	Nucleotide (s)
R	Purine nucleoside
rRNA	Ribosomal RNA
sRNA	Soluble RNA (now replaced by tRNA)
tRNA	Transfer RNA (formerly called as sRNA)
X	Any nucleoside
Y	Pyrimidine nucleoside